Genuine Recovery A Survivor Perspective

"GRASP offers important consideration of the nutritional and physical health status of an individual and its contribution to recovery and staying well."

Dr. Trudi Seneviratne, Consultant Psychiatrist, South London and Maudsley NHS Foundation Trust

"Umm Faruq's remarkable story of her strength and determination in exploring ways of maintaining her mental wellbeing without relapse for over nine years is both courageous and inspirational."

Haddy Quist, Nursing Team Leader, South London and Maudsley NHS Foundation Trust

"A magnificent text book manuscript; the message of the book is very clear, well argued and very well researched."

Gary Clarke, Mental Health Solicitor, Nathan Aaron Solicitors

"Umm Faruq makes the case that nutrition should be given a place alongside prescribed medication as a biological treatment for mental illness."

Anne Kendall, Head of Innovation Network, Rethink Mental Illness

"Reading GRASP has helped me; I am feeling a lot better and have hope for the future... I have control over my life again."

Amarjit Mlait

"The links between mind and body are so important and such a popular theme currently, so it feels the right time for such a book."

Alison Mohammed, Director of Regions, Rethink Mental Illness

Genuine Recovery A Survivor Perspective
Resolving Mental Illness

Umm Faruq
Survivor

978-0-9576774-1-8

Genuine Recovery a Survivor Perspective – Resolving Mental
Illness (paperback)

Published by Healthy 4 Real, London, United Kingdom.

Web address: www.healthy4real.com
Email: ummfaruq@o2.co.uk
Telephone: 07939468992

Disclaimer:

The contents of this book are meant to provide supplementary information and education pertaining to mental illness and mental health recovery. The information provided should not be construed as medical advice or used as a substitute for medical advice. The reader should seek proper medical advice in matters relating to his/her health and in particular with respect to any symptoms that may require diagnosis or medical attention.

Contents

For Mum

FOREWORD

With the World Health Organisation (WHO) estimating that by 2010 depression will be the number one cause of illness in the world, surpassing heart disease and cancer, it is imperative that policy makers, health professionals and patients work towards reducing the severity of the impact of mental ill health in our society. As a psychiatric nurse with years of experience working on acute wards, I often get disheartened by the futility of the revolving door system; patients come in and receive treatment, get better then discharged, get readmitted, treated, discharged and the whole cycle begins again. **Surely there has to be a more effective and cheaper means of working collaboratively to get people better for longer and maintaining a better quality of life after mental illness.**

In Umm Faruq's book, Genuine Recovery A Survivor Perspective (GRASP), she details her personal journey, her experiences and triumphs over adversities; the book is unapologetic and honest as it lays to bear every bit of science as well as the personal and social aspects of what makes us the people we are and why we may behave the way that we do. It is very much a resource/research book for everyone; service users, carers, mental health professionals and the general public.

GRASP takes a brave surge forward to answer often thought questions: is there a cure or management for mental and emotional health conditions? Is medication the only option? And where is the person behind the illness? Umm Faruq takes a pragmatic and practical, albeit solitary, stance to help herself and others, through her book, to find or discover their own recovery pathway towards positive mental health; chronicling her mental illness, treatment, recovery and empowerment; sharing details of what worked and how, using current evidence-based research to support her hypothesis.

Too often the Medical Model is bandied about as the only option for people experiencing severe emotional and mental health conditions. GRASP explores all the options with observations that are in line with the 2013 Croydon BME Forum report 'Mind the Gap' which states that medication seems often to be a point of tension for service users, who have expressed a need for better information regarding medications and side-effects; others expressing fears of becoming 'zombies' with the inability to communicate with others. Most particularly the exploration of nutrition as therapy, though it seems logical, is often not referred to nor sought by most medical professionals as part of the recovery model, which is a disservice to say the least to those on the recovery pathway.

Umm Faruq makes strong links with good nutrition, promoting collaborative self-recovery and self-management, and including a plethora of the most recent and relevant research papers to ensure the validity of her convictions. **This book will test your beliefs and your hard-held views, and it will take you to task whatever your stance is.** It gets technical in parts, but ride the waves as Umm Faruq takes you through the minutiae of cellular functions and physiological abilities. Bearing in mind the disclaimer that it is meant to provide the reader with 'supplementary information and education', GRASP is a no-holds-barred book; one for all seasons, and can be referred to time and time again.

GRASP will benefit countless people and give some hope that having a mental health condition does not mean you lose the right or power to live a healthy and fulfilling life. The writer was determined to share her experiences, now it is left for those that read this book to make their own way to autonomy, empowerment and recovery.

RISQ ANIMASAUN
BME MENTAL HEALTH COMMUNITY DEVELOPMENT
WORKER, CROYDON BME FORUM

INTRODUCTION

First and foremost, all praise is due to God All-Mighty (Allaah [Glorified and Exalted]), for guiding me to His religion Islam. Being a Muslim, I believe that my religious faith (belief and practice) has provided me with the basis to clearly distinguish truth from falsehood, which has helped in restoring my sanity, health and wellbeing. I thank God for giving me the presence of mind and ability to write this book which you now hold.

A Brief Background to the Writing of This Book

For over 10 years, I have been thinking and talking about writing a book on mental health recovery, but would only keep gathering information through research and not actually start writing the book. However, nothing happens before the time is right.

Looking back, the time was certainly NOT right. Even though I was on the road to recovery, I now realise that I was still not quite well enough (plus I was still very angry about the way I had been treated in hospital). Also, to be quite honest, I wasn't even fully convinced that I would be able stay out of hospital long enough to complete my journey, let alone convince others that I had indeed fully recovered. Whilst coming off medication, I lived in fear of relapsing to the extent where others would find out, which could mean ending up on another section. I had no choice but to pretend as though I was still taking my medication and would collect my prescriptions as usual.

I also acknowledged within myself (through constant self-monitoring) that I still had a lot more learning and experimental self-treatment to do before celebrating recovery. My goal was to learn and understand as much as possible about my illness and find ways to help myself overcome the horrors I was experiencing (such as psychosis, losing the sense of my own identity, hearing voices, delusions, paranoia and so on).

On one occasion my son and son-in-law came to my flat and I ignored the door. I did not answer my phone either, because I knew that if they saw the terrible state I was in they would not have understood what I was doing (or agree with my coming off medication) and would have most likely contacted my doctor. I also would not have been able to explain myself or convince them that I was busy trying to cure my illness. If they only saw how I looked and the way I was behaving... Can you imagine how they might have responded to that statement?

Even though I realised that my son (in particular) was beside himself with worry, I knew it would only be worse if he saw me, so I ignored the door and his calls through the letterbox. I certainly wasn't going to let anyone ruin my efforts to recover; I believed that I was making some progress and just had to ride this one through.

In spite of these experiences, I certainly did not believe that I had to remain on medication for life, but I still had no real evidence, information or knowledge to prove otherwise. Nevertheless, this did not deter me from trying to help myself. In fact, it was my view that because it was *my* sanity and *my* health that was at stake, then it ought to be *my* decision on what was best for me, anyway. So, I made up my mind that I was not going to listen to what anyone else had to say (regardless of who they were: friend or foe), and I was prepared to learn the hard way if it came down to it.

My self-induced challenge was made even more difficult and complex by having to find ways to cope with withdrawal symptoms from the medication as well as the illness. It was very hard work trying to distinguish/separate the source of one set of symptoms from the other – was it the withdrawal or the illness?

Most of the time the withdrawal symptoms resembled full blown psychosis and paranoia, but because I had experienced those types of withdrawal symptoms before (in my previous attempts to get off medication) I recognised that I had to replace the medication with an alternative to get through the bad patch. I chose to use nutritional and herbal treatments to address and ease the impact of the withdrawal. At the same time, I knew that I could not dare let anyone see me in the state I was because I would have been taken back to hospital (most likely placed on a section and forced to take more medication).

After recovering, I spent the next 10 years researching and educating myself. I also took some professional training courses, studying Clinical Nutrition and Clinical Herbalism. I then used what I had learnt to prepare nutritional/herbal formulas for myself, testing to see if they worked or not.

You may have figured out for yourself by now that I can be a very determined person... one who is not prepared give up without a fight!

The key driving force behind this determination was to learn the truth and be able to help my mother, myself and others suffering from severe mental illnesses. The question I was determined to get the answers to was: Is it really true that because I have a severe mental disorder, and a family history of this disorder, this means I have to remain on anti-psychotic medications for the rest of my life (just like my mother and my brother)?

How I Lost My Mother to the Mental Health System

I had witnessed my mother go through a lot a suffering, due to her mental illness (as well as not being listened to in her refusal of medications). I desperately wanted help her but had no idea what mental illness was like and what she might have been going though. I wanted to learn, understand and to find an answer. Most of all, I wanted my mum back. This was during the period before my own experience of mental illness.

My mother had been in and out of psychiatric hospitals for almost as long as I could remember. She was not happy with having to be forced to take medication and would have preferred, and been much happier, to take something more natural to avoid the side-effects and allow her to retain her independence.

Unfortunately, my mother had no choice: she was forced to comply and to this day no other treatment options (sans medication) have been offered nor any choice given.

Many years ago, my father (who is now deceased) and I tried to exercise our rights under the Mental Health Act (as nearest relatives) to have my mother discharged from section and returned home. Unfortunately, this failed because my father was promptly displaced as the nearest relative and we were left powerless to change the situation.

Now, after many years of being on a variety of anti-psychotics, my mother's mental state has deteriorated... far worse than she ever was in the very beginning, to the point where she has now become totally institutionalised. My mother has never been able to get back to a point where she is able to leave hospital and be home again. I believe that the forced anti-psychotics and lack of alternative/choice caused me to lose my mother.

This negative outcome that my mother has had only served to make me even more determined not to have a similar outcome, and I certainly do not relish the idea that other members of my family/relatives (or anyone else) may be doomed to a similar negative fate with no opportunity for meaningful treatment choices/options.

So, now I have had my questions answered, and now I know the truth with certainty: there are alternative ways for taking care of and treating people like my mother (who are unhappy with taking medications). I also know with certainty that a person with serious mental illness does not have to be on medication for their entire life to get well and remain well, even those with a family history of mental illness.

I acknowledge that in some cases an individual may need to be on medication for a long period or maybe even for life. Nevertheless, a range of alternative treatment options/choices should be made available, especially for those individuals that are refusing/unhappy with taking anti-psychotics.

"In our haste to 'fix' people with schizophrenia, we suffocate them and don't allow them to learn and adjust to living with it themselves – which is entirely possible for most. The system itself becomes the barrier to this individual growth and adjustment; personal recovery becomes elusive."
(Rethink Mental Illness, 2012).

"We should respect an individual's right to decide and inform themselves around issues relating to their own mental health."
(Rethink Mental Illness, 2012)

A Glimpse at My Past and Journey to Recovery

I had my first admission to a psychiatric unit round about the early 1980's. I remember being aware that something had changed in my perception of myself and the way I was seeing the world and other people, however, I had no idea that I was experiencing a mental breakdown. Thinking back, I remember wondering why everyone around me seemed to be behaving differently, and I saw this as them not realising that I was having a "special" experience which they were not able to understand. At one point I remember thinking that at last I had gotten in touch with my real self (or true calling); I believed that the real me had been trapped/imprisoned inside somewhere. In a number of ways the experience felt very good to me (initially), so I welcomed it and didn't feel the need to do anything about it.

Delusions

Things took a turn for the worse: I was not able to sleep for several nights and I started feeling very tormented. During this period I experienced a number of nightmarish hallucinations, including seeing an image of a person appearing in my room through my bedroom wall, which made it even more impossible for me to sleep and I also became extremely paranoid.

In another of my delusional, psychotic episodes, I believed I was a witness to my own murder. I remember lying on the floor in my flat, paralysed with fear because I could feel heavy blows to my head from a large, blunt object; I believed that someone had entered my flat and was bludgeoning me to death. At the same time I was also convinced that I had a special ability that would allow me to come back from the dead and give witness to my murder. I believed that I possessed the 'all-seeing eye' and that a number of people were out to get me because of it.

When I was taken to hospital (by my father) I just could not understand why I was being detained. At one point I thought that they were only pretending to be nursing staff but were really part of the 'This is Your Life' team (a 1970s TV show hosted by Eamonn Andrews). I believed they wanted to surprise me with the 'Big Red Book'. I still believed that I had come back from the dead and wanted to let everyone know. I also believed this to be the reason that no-one seemed to understand what I was saying. At other times I believed that some people did indeed know that I had come back from the dead, but were keeping it a secret because if everyone knew they might try to capture me and keep me for some kind of experimental research.

Paranoia

Because of the way the hospital staff were behaving and looking at me, I started to become suspicious of their actions. I started to believe that the hospital staff had been set up to capture me. This caused me to feel extreme panic and desperation to get away; like a wild animal caught in a trap. I was determined to leave the hospital. As you can probably tell, by that stage I was becoming overwhelmed by paranoia and intense feelings of dread. There are no words to describe or express what this experience was like, only those who have lived with the experience of extreme paranoia will be able to relate to this.

I was absolutely petrified of staff or doctors coming anywhere near me because I did not trust them and I believed that they were plotting to jump and trap me. So, I kept moving around (trying to keep them in sight and not turning my back) and at times shouting at them to stay away from me. One member of staff ignored my shouts to stay away and approached me anyway. I head butted him, and at that point I was rushed by a number staff and doctors. In my mind I believed that they were intent on doing serious harm to me. I was angry and put up a vicious struggle, trying to break free from them. Eventually, I was pinned down and given an injection which knocked me out. To this day I have no idea what I was injected with, all I know is that I was out like a light.

This admission marked the beginning of a number of subsequent admissions to psychiatric hospital. Over that period of time I experienced a number of different manifestations/presentations of mental illness and was given different diagnoses such as Schizophrenia, Paranoid Schizophrenia, and Manic Depression.

Coming Off Medication

The admission/readmission scenario repeated itself on several occasions, and the side-effects I experienced each time from the medications were horrendous, to say the least.

During all of this, I had firmly made up my mind that I would take myself off medication as soon as the first opportunity arrived. I was convinced that there had to be a better way; and I was determined to find it; even if it was the last thing I ever did.

I was well aware, however, that I would not have had the consent or support of my consultant or family to stop taking the medications. After all, I had already been told that I would have to be on medication for life and that my illness was linked to a family history of mental illness. What this meant was that I had no choice but to go it alone, and to keep my decision to stop medication a secret from everyone – which was exactly what I did.

My first few attempts at stopping medication were a real disaster, to say the least; the withdrawal effects of the medication were even worse than the illness. Before I knew it... you guessed it! I was sectioned again and forced with more medication, being told that my 'relapse' was because I was not taking it.

Nevertheless, I was not about to give up. As soon as I was discharged from hospital, I developed another plan: this time I decided to come off the medications at a slower pace, as well as learn about alternative measures to take to stop myself from relapsing.

This marked the beginning of my journey of research, self-education and learning, guided by some of the tremendous insights that I had gained though my own lived experience of severe mental disorder. Learning from the many different manifestations and presentations helped me to identify a range of triggers and, therefore, how to address them at an early stage.

Knowledge Truly Is Power!

Writing this book is a way for me to celebrate and share my success and learning with others.

This book is not intended to say to anyone that they should stop taking medications, because what I learnt is that there is a place for medication, which is, primarily, over a short term and during major crisis. I certainly do not agree that medication should be over-relied upon (or that a person should be forced into compliance) as the solution to severe mental illness, especially over long-term. I do strongly believe that the goal should be to reduce and eventually take individuals off medication, especially if they are voicing objections and concerns about having to take them.

The core message of this book is that whether or not a person is currently taking or is to remain on medication, essential nutrition has an intricate and overarching role to play in achieving successful recovery outcomes (especially from those conditions related to comorbidity).

I am happy to say that my last admission to a psychiatric unit took place in 2001 (almost 13 years ago to date).

<u>Choice and Clarity of Decision Making is Dependent Upon Knowledge</u>

Is there any evidence of a need for more treatment options/choices?

Excerpts from the Rethink Mental Illness Schizophrenia Commission Report 2012: The abandoned illness.

For many the treatment route using powerful chemical interventions is flawed. Often, the consequences of illness combined with medication do not have a positive outcome. They lose everything of the person they were before and make little or no progress towards wellness. A carer at the Rethink AGM said:

"[Of her loved one] He had a great life before, then was completely transformed into someone else by what had happened to him and the system – now he languishes in a care home."

Clearly, for some, just offering medication is not appropriate as a viable solution to their mental distress or experience. They need something else as a workable alternative, and all the evidence I have seen supports this. We need to acknowledge one simple truth: medication for psychosis does not work for all.

The theme of side-effects and their debilitating consequences is really the main sticking point with medication. Chronic weight gain, sexual dysfunction, numbing of the spirit, dietary problems, sleep problems, and more, can all make life unbearable for many. It directly affects compliance with the whole medical regime – many would simply rather be unwell than go through all of that.

"We have a massive scientific reliance on medication for therapeutic effects which do not cure people and often produce distressing side-effects. If compared to other health conditions, would this even be allowed?" (Diana Rose)

"I was told that I would have to be on medication for the rest of my life. I have been free of medication and free of symptoms for 12 years. Mental illness can be dealt with in many other ways." (Louise Gillett)

(Rethink Mental Illness, 2012)

This book contains a number of relevant information compiled from various articles that are freely available on the Internet. Where possible I have provided references for these. By sharing this information gained from evidence-based research over many years, including insights from my own lived experience and from my work as a mental health professional, this book is aimed at empowering those suffering from mental illness.

I believe others can, through reading this book, gain insight to assist with making informed decisions about their own mental health treatment/self-management. I believe that the information in this book will support the case for working collaboratively on achieving the best care/recovery outcomes.

The information in this book will help to increase insightful knowledge about the importance of meaningful treatment options, such as nutritional therapy, to build physical and mental resilience; leading to recovery, sustained mental health and holistic wellbeing.

This book is for you whether you are a:

- Patient/service user
- Parent
- Responsible clinician
- Family member of someone with a mental disorder
- Carer of someone with a mental disorder
- Professional working in the caring field
- Outreach professional
- An employer (with staff who have/had mental health problems)
- A friend

- Someone who just wants to learn more and to educate themselves
- Someone who believes that prevention is better than cure
- Service providers/stakeholders
- Commissioners of service
- Mental or physical health educator

As you continue to read though the pages of this book, you will gain knowledge to better understand about the numerous ways nutrition therapy can not only aid successful recovery, but also influence our genetic expression (in terms of health or disease) and the rate at which we age biologically.

PART ONE
Illness: The Mind-Body Connection

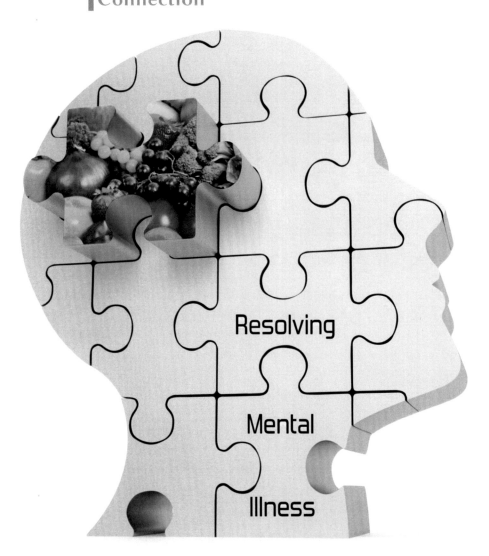

Resolving

Mental

Illness

THERE ARE ALWAYS terms and labels for everything, but I would call it nutritional therapy, because I've had to use nutrition as a therapy for myself in order to function.

When I was taking medication for my mental illness, I couldn't think very well – which was one of the side-effects, and was why I hated it so much; my thinking ability was hampered and I struggled to gain focus. After stopping the medication, however, even speaking about the mental illness would make me feel as if I was going to break down; the whole body system is involved in the withdrawal, and I had to recognise that I was going through a traumatic experience.

I realised that I had to deal with those symptoms as well as my illness, and nutrition was the way I did it – making sure that I had taken in enough water, vitamins and sleep. Obviously, my religion played a very big role in my recovery, because not only did it help me to focus but also to know that I was not alone in terms of the things I was able to accomplish. That's quite a big area of my life now.

For me there is a genetic tendency towards mental illness, and even though I've used nutrition to become well, I know that the vulnerability will remain there. At times I may feel myself going a bit, but I know what to do now.

1   NUTRITION AND HEALTH

One in four people will suffer from some kind of mental illness during their life.

Nutrition has a profound impact on both our mental and physical health. Even so, it's only more recently that scientists have started to conduct research into this relationship.

There are many things we can do to help promote our mental health and one example is having good nutrition.

Nutrition is what fuels the human body. It makes up our cells, tissues, organs and everything that makes us alive and human. Nutrition from the foods we eat is used as a source of energy for survival. But nutrition plays one more important role: it helps the body recover.

Good nutrition is vital for brain function and it also minimises the risk of cardiovascular disease, diabetes and other lifestyle diseases.

Generally, people with serious mental illness have been found to have poorer nutrition than the general population.

This proves that the food we eat goes further than our physical health; it can also affect how we feel and how we behave, and it goes without saying that taking care of mental health is hugely important.

Diet, or to be precise - a bad diet, can affect several areas of mental health that can lead to the following problems:

- Depression
- Mood swings/disorders
- Stress
- Seasonal Affective Disorder (SAD)
- Panic attacks
- Memory problems

For example, a person who has missed a meal can often be easily distracted and irritable. If this is prolonged, energy levels can experience a huge dip, leading to changes in hormone levels and a lack of nutrients being transported to certain areas of the body, all of which can eventually influence mental health.

Nutritional imbalances play a critical role in mental health. Many emotional and behavioural symptoms and disorders have, at their root, nutritional and biochemical imbalances that either cause or aggravate them.

As the role of nutrition is increasingly identified as an important factor in the acquisition of mental well-being, and as mental health clients present with more physical illness than the general population, some in the field have identified:

"an urgent need for effective nutrition and exercise interventions for the users of mental health services."
(Isenring, 2008).

This is no call to a cursory glance at a client's dietary intake, as the expertise needed to affect a complete understanding of the physical and mental processes involved in the body's assimilation of food is:

"a speciality in itself."
(Quinn, 2009).

Appropriate nutrition is essential for:

• The growth and development of brains and bodies.
• Building, maintaining, fuelling and repairing of EVERY cell in EVERY part of the brain and body.

At least 39 essential nutrients MUST be provided by our food.   These include vitamins and minerals, essential amino acids, and omega-3 and Omega-6 fatty acids.   Many of these essential nutrients are lacking from modern diets.

Individual differences affect dietary requirements – specific nutrients may be needed in unusually high quantities or there may be allergies or intolerances to certain foods. These individual differences in physical make up and – by extension – nutritional requirements form the basis of what is called our 'Biochemical Individuality'.

WHAT WE'VE GOT to understand is that our bodies are made up of a number of different organs and cells and they all have different jobs to perform. When it comes to nutrients we need all different types; the main thing is that our bodies need to be balanced and that balance isn't standard for everybody.

Just as we're individuals in terms of our preferences – some people may like apples, some may not and may prefer oranges – we are also individuals in terms of our genetic make-up. And just as on the outside we all look different, inside our genes express differently also.

This biochemical individuality can be seen in effect when medication is prescribed. A person may be given something like olanzapine (an atypical anti-psychotic) and then it's trial and error because some people may show progress whilst others become worse. Then they'll be taken off that or given something to deal with side effects – which are not standard either. With everything you'll find that people will have slightly different reactions or maybe even opposing reactions.

Or a person may have a genetic tendency towards a particular condition – diabetes or Alzheimer's for example. This just means that they have to acknowledge their weakness in that area and make a special effort in terms of their nutrition.

Biochemical individuality refers to the unique nutritional needs each person has, based on their genetics, lifestyle, and environmental exposure to various stresses. It is a critical reason for certain nutritional imbalances that often lead to emotional and mental problems. Biochemistry is a complex web of interactions that controls the way your body uses amino acids, vitamins, minerals, carbohydrates, and fats for all your bodily functions. Each one of us has a biochemistry that's unique, and along with our internal environment, it determines the strengths and weaknesses in our health. We can see this uniqueness by the variations in genes, by the preferences for different diets, and in the way people might have a similar diagnosis but have different underlying or contributing factors to it. Those characteristics make someone who they are, and this is true for more or less everything; from the way we look on the outside all the way down to our cells.

There is no one size fits all! Everyone is unique in terms of their biochemistry; **one man's meat is another man's poison.**

For your biochemistry to balance properly, your body requires the right amounts and proportions of nutrients. The amount of certain nutrients that the 'average person' requires may not be the optimal amount that *you* need for good health.

Symptoms of disease can occur in response to problems with biochemical processes. Depression provides a good example. The body requires certain nutrients in order to manufacture mood-regulating hormones (serotonin, dopamine and epinephrine). For these hormones to be properly manufactured, your body needs the amino acids Phenylalanine and Tryptophan; vitamins B_3 and B_6; and the minerals Iron and Copper. Low levels of these nutrients (the raw materials needed to manufacture hormones), can induce depression.

People may become deficient in required nutrients because they don't get enough of the specific vitamins, minerals and amino acids in their diet, or their unique biochemistry may simply require additional amounts of one or more nutrients for the biochemical pathway to function properly.

Today we live in a stressed-out world, and an increasing body of research suggests that our hyper-vigilant lifestyle is severely impacting on the health of our bodies. Daily stressors and emotional upsets are constantly activating the part of our neuroendocrine system responsible for stress response and the regulation of many of our bodily processes: the Hypothalamic-Pituitary-Adrenal (HPA) axis. This causes emotional and physical disharmony that triggers major illness such as cardio vascular and digestive issues, depression, and glucose/insulin resistance. Further, these stressors are not released from the body (as they would be in a fight or flight situation) and can build up to become chronic fears and concerns.

Autonomic System Regulation

Most people are familiar with the central nervous system (CNS), which consists of the brain and the spinal cord. Another, less well known but equally important, part of the nervous system is the peripheral nervous system (PNS).

As its name suggests, the PNS carries information back and forth between the control centre (the brain) and the periphery. It communicates to the brain what is going on in the environment outside the body via the senses: hearing, touch, taste and smell (the eyes are unusual in that they are directly part of the brain and so are classed as part of the CNS).

The PNS also communicates to the brain what is happening in other parts of the body. So, for instance, it controls and monitors heartbeat, blood pressure and the release of hormones from glands such as the thyroid, pituitary and pancreas. It does so autonomously – in other words, independently of our will. This is why this part of the PNS is called the autonomic nervous system (ANS).

To illustrate just how much we depend on both nervous systems, let's go through how we start the day.

Several hours before we awake, our PNS is monitoring body functions and communicating to the brain (CNS) that we are soon to wake up (this is called our circadian clock, activated by light and dark). As we awake by the sound of the alarm (hearing – PNS), we open our eyes and register our surroundings (sight – CNS). We register the scent of coffee and toast from the kitchen (smell – PNS) and get out of bed; our feet touch the floor and we stand up (touch, balance – PNS). We eat breakfast (smell, taste, digestion – PNS), and so on. All the while, the autonomic part of our peripheral nervous system has been monitoring heartbeat, blood pressure and hormone levels, and we have used our brain (CNS) to interpret those vital signals.

Furthermore, when the body needs nourishment, neurotransmitters are released. One neurotransmitter called Neuropeptide Y (NPY) is instrumental in sending messages to various parts of the brain. Information is fed into the brain through the senses. What is heard, felt, tasted, seen, or smelt is detected by receptors in or on the body and sent to the brain through sensory neurons. The brain decides what to do with the information from the senses and tells the body how to respond by sending out messages via motor neurons. For example, if a person puts his or her hand near something hot, the sense of touch tells the brain about the heat and the brain sends a message to the muscles of the arm to move the hand away.

Biochemical Individuality and the Autonomic Nervous System

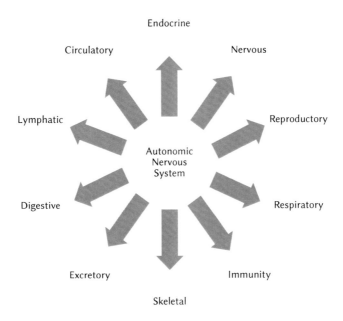

Endocrine

Circulatory

Nervous

Lymphatic

Reproductory

Autonomic
Nervous
System

Digestive

Respiratory

Excretory

Immunity

Skeletal

There are two main factors that tie into your nutritional uniqueness or biochemical individuality. One is based on your ANS regulation. The other is to do with oxidation, which will be discussed later in this chapter. From the diagram above, you can see that the ANS is the master regulator of your body. If there is a function going on in your body, it is tied directly into the ANS function. All the bodily systems, from the circulatory system to the excretory system, are regulated by the ANS.

What most people don't understand is that there are two main divisions to the ANS, and these are significantly influenced by nutrition. If we look at these two divisions, we're looking at:

- **Parasympathetic** – This is like the brakes; it slows you down and relaxes you; it controls all your body functions that work in a relaxed state.
- **Sympathetic** – This is like the gas; it speeds you up; it controls everything to do with the **'fight or flight'** response.

A dynamic balance needs to exist between the two divisions of the autonomic nervous system so that they can continuously make fine adjustments.

As pointed out above, your parasympathetic nervous system's function is more of the relaxed side of the nervous system; it is the aspect of the nervous system that allows your bodily functions to actually occur without you having to think about it.

There is not one person in existence that has to think for their kidneys to function. There is not one person in existence that has to think for their heart to function or for them to breathe or for any of those bodily functions to actually occur. All of this is due to the parasympathetic function of the ANS.

Now, the opposite, which is your sympathetic nervous system, and is referred to as the 'fight or flight' aspect, kicks in not only when you're in a truly life or death situation, but also whenever there is a stress response that's created based on perceptions in the mind. Once stress is created, whatever it is that creates the stress, the 'fight or flight' response is going to trigger a sympathetic response.

Most of us can recognise stress as a part of our lives and the lives of other people we know.

But what has long gone unrecognised is that you can actually create sympathetic or parasympathetic dominance by eating food. For example, an individual may already be sympathetically dominant and then eat the types of food that influences further sympathetic dominance.

The problem with that is, the body normally needs to function in a parasympathetic state because that's when the body repairs and maintains itself. The body is **anabolic** when the nervous system is in a parasympathetic dominant state and **catabolic** when the nervous system is in a sympathetic dominant state.

If you are anabolic, your body is able to repair itself; you will have good absorption and elimination; you will sleep well and wake rested; you will feel relaxed and energetic; your muscles, bones, joints, hair, and nails will be strong and healthy, and your cuts, strains, and injuries will heal readily.

If you are catabolic; your body will be unable to heal itself, you will have digestive problems (heartburn, indigestion) and poor elimination; you will sleep fitfully and wake up tired, and you will have joint and muscle aches and pains.

So these factors are amongst the keys that are tied into your nutritional uniqueness. The important thing to bear in mind is that your goal is to get a good balanced relationship between the parasympathetic and the sympathetic nervous systems, and this is primarily achieved with nutrition. So why is this balance so important for mental health?

The Autonomic Nervous System and Stress Response

Mental health is intimately connected with physical health and behaviour. Whatever impacts us mentally also impacts us physically and vice versa.

Emotional challenges and physiological experiences are often described in terms of the word 'stress'.

Stress involves two-way communication between the brain and the cardiovascular, immune, and other systems via neural and endocrine mechanisms.

The brain is the organ of the body that interprets experiences as threatening or nonthreatening and which determines the behavioural and physiological responses to each situation.

A hallmark of the stress response is the activation of the ANS.

The nervous system, like all tissues of the body, is composed of cells. There are two major types of nerve cell: **glial cells** and **neurons**.

Glial cells are the brain's support network. They help maintain the environment surrounding the neurons, and are responsible for Myelin (a fatty substance that insulates nerve cells in order to speed up communications).

Neurons, on the other hand, are the messengers of the brain. Their job is to take information and move it as quickly as possible from one cell to another. Neurons consist of a cell body with protrusions – short dendrites and longer axons. The axons of motor neurons carry electrical information away from the brain via the spinal cord to the muscles and organs in the periphery. Sensory neurons transmit information in the opposite direction from the periphery via the spinal cord to the brain. Based on this information the brain then decides what action to take.

So, neurons do the job of thinking, computing, remembering, organising, sensing and activating. There are billions of neurons in the brain, sending and receiving information that make up our thoughts, control our behaviour, regulate our bodies and much more.

How are all these neurons able to communicate? They communicate through a combination of electrical and chemical signals.

When a neuron is activated, an electric signal is sent from one end of the neuron to the other. As it gets closer to the other side, this neuron can split into many fine branches. At the end of these branches, chemicals called neurotransmitters are stored in specialised swellings.

When the electrical impulse reaches these swellings, it signals the release of neurotransmitters into the space between the two neurons. This space is called a synapse.

The outer surface of the other neuron is covered with receptors. Neurotransmitters cross the synapse and fit into receptors (like keys fitting a lock). When this connection is made, it signals the next neuron.

Some neurotransmitters will tell the next neuron to create an electrical impulse. Others will prevent a neuron from creating an electrical impulse.

The average neuron forms about 1000 connections with other neurons, which means there are lots of different chemicals floating around in the synapse.

So, how does each neuron know what to do when its receptors are activated?

The receptors on a neuron's surface will only connect with a specific type of neurotransmitter that has the right chemical shape. Neurotransmitters that do not have the right set will not bind to the receptor and therefore will not cause a response. And a neuron will only respond when enough neurotransmitters have fit into its receptors.

Whether the neuron sends a signal, depends on the amount and type of neurotransmitter that have connected to its receptors.

Once the neurotransmitters have done their job, the majority of them return to the neuron that sent them, clearing the synapse for the next signal. This is called reuptake.

Even though this process seems complicated, the entire information transmission process occurs in the brain and other parts of the nervous system within a matter of seconds.

So, the ANS is activated in response to stress – a mental perception causing a physical response.

Don't forget the ANS is responsible for certain reactions – for example to do with fear and life saving responses i.e. breathing, sleep and system regulation, and each person will differ slightly in terms of their automatic bodily responses. But when we are stressed, the ANS becomes overactive, and when this happens increased oxidation inevitably follows. How this happens is that when a person is stressed it stimulates the person into action and that is the sympathetic side of the ANS being stimulated. So a person will breathe faster, their heart rate will be elevated, and sugars will be released into the body to provide energy to the muscles, etc. As that happens, oxidation (put simply – nutrient conversion into fuel) will also be occurring at an increased rate. Being aware of your nutrition is important so that you can increase certain foods and decrease certain other foods to help balance your body's sympathetic/parasympathetic state.

Acidity is a similar state to oxidation as it starts breakdown processes in the body. Anything that causes cell breakdown can be referred to as oxidation, free radicalisation, etc. They are slightly different processes but they ultimately they do the same thing – cause a breakdown of cells – and as you know, cells make up tissues and tissues make up organs. So this is not something to be taken lightly because if cells are being broken down at an increased rate then eventually an organ could fail. Why? Because organs are made of tissues which are made up of cells, thus cells make you up as an organism. If our diets are lacking in the nutrients required to repair the damage of over-oxidation, this eventual organ failure is a likelihood.

All the time the body is trying to regulate these processes. The hypothalamus is responsible for a lot of regulation – sleep, temperature, hormone release, etc. – and it works very closely with the nervous system. This will be discussed further in chapter 15: *Sleep*.

Oxidation and Energy

As mentioned earlier, the other main factor that ties in to your nutritional uniqueness is related to oxidation. Your oxidation rate is the speed at which your body can process the food and nutrients you consume and eventually convert this into energy. So what's happening is: you're converting carbohydrates into energy through a system of glycolysis, eventually ending up in the citric acid cycle. This is basically the conversion of carbohydrates into useable energy.

We experience hunger to produce energy, NOT to fill our stomach.

Often we can fill our stomachs and still not produce energy. Remember, you're always hungry to produce energy, so when you consume the proper foods, you are addressing your nutritional uniqueness and need for energy.

As a result the trigger for hunger will be cut off substantially quicker within your meal, than if you're eating the wrong foods.

For example, those of you who enjoy eating pizza will probably notice that you really gorge yourself on pizza. You can generally eat much more pizza than you could with most other foods. The big reason for this is that pizza does not have a high level of nutrition, so you typically will eat pizza until you're physically full. You actually reach the point where you have filled your stomach. This will now cause the body to release the trigger to stop eating and you will stop eating.

But here's what typically happens next: because of the lack of available nutrients within the pizza, you will stop eating because you feel physically filled in the stomach, but you still never really produce the energy that your body demanded in the first place. This has an impact on your body, so what happens at that point to most people in this position, is that they get the urge to eat something sweet; we all know that sugar is a 'quick fix' for energy.

So, when you haven't produced the energy that your body needs from your meal, yet you've still filled your stomach to the point where the trigger for hunger has been shut down, you will get a sweet craving.

This is a cycle that happens time and time again within the western culture, and it's really a cycle that eventually leads to chronic illness and disease.

Every type of nutritional uniqueness needs macronutrients and micronutrients. In other words, we all need varying amounts of fruits and vegetables, carbohydrates, fats and proteins. And even for vegetarians, it's essential to get some levels of protein by perhaps focusing on the correct combinations of plant-based proteins.

Basically, each person needs to have variety based on their own individual and unique needs, their environment and what goes on in their daily lives.

Oxidation, Energy and Mental Health

"Since the brain and the nervous system use proportionately more energy than any other of the body's organs, when there is a dysfunction in the energy cycles, the first adverse effects are found in one's thinking, feeling and behaviour."
(Watson, 1979).

Glucose is one vital fuel for the brain. The brain's activities rely heavily on glucose for energy (Laughlin, 2004); (Seisjo, 1978); (Weiss, 1978).

The metabolisation of glucose from the bloodstream allows each brain region to carry out its given functions (McNay, McCarty, & Gold, 2001); (Reivich & Alavi, 1983).

Even though nearly all of the brain's activities consume some glucose, most cognitive processes are relatively unaffected by subtle or minor fluctuations in glucose levels within the normal or healthy range. Controlled, effortful processes that rely on executive function, however, are unlike most other cognitive processes in that they seem highly susceptible to normal fluctuations in glucose.

For instance, low glucose has been linked with impaired performance on complex (as opposed to simple) reaction time tasks (Owens & Benton, 1994). One study found that low glucose was associated with poor performance on a driving simulation task, but only toward the end of the task when participants were fatigued and the task was most demanding (Benton, 1990).

Low glucose, therefore, seems to impair controlled or effortful processes but not the simpler or automatic processes, most likely because controlled processes require more glucose than automatic processes (Fairclough & Houston, 2004).

The oxidation of metabolic fuels (protein, carbohydrate and fat) produces energy in the form of Adenosine Triphosphate (ATP). This energy is used to drive chemical reactions.

The production of energy (ATP) from our food involves two major components: an intact energy pathway and a balanced metabolic or oxidative rate.

Oxidation is actually the process by which certain elements in the body combine with oxygen to release energy from food and is actually the chemical process of burning.

In other words, food burns to produce energy!

For example, when you burn a piece of wood, the wood is being oxidised. You are causing the wood to combine rapidly with oxygen to cause a high-intensity energy release. Oxidation can occur at different speeds. The human Oxidation Rate is the rate at which the body's cells are "burning" their fuel, or food.

ATP is the universal currency of energy in the cell. The body requires a continual supply of energy for its functions, such as:

- Muscle contraction
- Biosynthesis of proteins, carbohydrates and fats
- Active transport of molecules and ions across cell membranes

How does this tie into biochemical individuality?

There are four main classifications to describe the different rates at which people release energy from their food:

1. **A Slow Oxidiser** releases energy too slowly. He/she is like a wood stove whose fire is too small to heat up the room. To create health, they must speed up their metabolic furnace, i.e. oxidation rate must be INCREASED.
2. **A Fast Oxidiser** releases energy too quickly. He/she is like a wood stove that is burning too fast, overheating the room (body), and running out of fuel. Oxidation rate must be DECREASED.
3. **A Mixed-Oxidiser** has an erratic metabolism: sometimes it is too fast, sometimes too slow. To create more energy, a Mixed Oxidizer must STABILISE his/her oxidation rate.
4. **The Balanced Oxidiser** has the most EFFICIENT metabolism. It is neither too fast nor too slow. His/her system produces the

maximum amount of usable human energy. To bring a person to a state of balanced oxidation is the main goal of Nutritional Balancing.

A slow oxidiser has higher than normal calcium and magnesium levels, and lower than normal sodium and potassium levels. The thyroid and adrenal glands are underactive. Slow oxidation is basically a defensive holding pattern. The body is in a state of defence against stress; it has gone into a protective shell to ward off any demands on its mineral reserves.

The super slow oxidiser feels weak and tired. He/she is lethargic, doesn't like to start new things and is too tired to even care about things happening around them.

The fast oxidiser has lower than normal calcium and magnesium levels and higher than normal sodium and potassium levels. The thyroid and adrenal glands are overactive. The fast oxidiser does not give in to fatigue – he attacks it. They go into an over-burn so that the same pace can be maintained. The fast oxidiser needs stress to keep them going; if they did not stay hyped-up and keyed-up, they would collapse. That's why the fast oxidiser goes to pieces when things become mundane. When things are too quiet, their organs don't get the stimulation they need to carry on.

In the mixed oxidiser, one of the energy-producing glands (thyroid or adrenals) is fast while the other is slow. These two glands are out of sync. Mixed oxidisers are on an energy roller-coaster, having periods of energy spurts followed by precipitous collapses. A mixed oxidiser will have a tendency towards either fast or slow oxidation. The further this trend is towards fast, the more pronounced will be the roller-coaster effect. A mixed oxidiser who leans towards slow oxidation will probably not notice much fluctuation at all.

The balanced oxidiser, the most powerful of all oxidation types, has an oxidation rate that is just right; not too fast and not too slow. Balanced oxidisers are the most productive people of all. Their bodies provide them with a steady, controlled, constant release of usable energy. They are happy, content, open and uncomplicated. They possess an inner calm and steadiness.

Conditions associated with slow oxidation are, for example:

- Fatigue
- Adrenal Burnout
- Depression
- Migraines
- Allergies
- Asthma
- Acne
- Constipation
- Weight Gain
- Diabetes
- Heart Disease, and
- Arthritis.

These are just a few common conditions which are often associated with slow oxidation.

It is important to note that all of the above conditions can also occur in fast oxidisers, only they are caused by different biochemical reactions.

Oxidation always takes place – cells are breaking down all the time, repairing, dying, and the body is excreting dead cells etc. – however the rate of oxidation will depend on that person's own biochemical individuality as well as what is happening in their life. If they're under stress, oxidation speeds up. If they are sick, oxidation will also take place more rapidly. If a person isn't getting enough sleep, oxidation will increase.

So what's the problem with increased oxidation?

When increased oxidation is taking place, glucose build-up in the system occurs. This is because the body is unable to use the sugars in the body as appropriately as it should. People can thus end up with diabetes due to stress, and other degenerative diseases. When there is glucose in the system, glucose molecules attach themselves like glue to proteins and lipids; a process called glycation. If, however, there is insufficient movement going on due to excess glycation, and the glucose energy isn't being used, this causes further deterioration and breakdown, leading to conditions such as Alzheimer's, dementia, Parkinson's, impaired thinking and impaired function, etc. if left un-checked. So, excess sugar in the body is not a good situation –

whether this is by direct sugar intake, by the intake of foods that break down very rapidly into glucose, or by stress – causing increased oxidation.

Importance of Balancing Glucose and Insulin for Health

Therefore, one of the most important things we can do to maintain health is to keep our glucose and insulin levels as low as possible. The reason for this is that when glucose levels are higher in the blood, we undergo a rate of glycation that is much faster than normal.

The problem with high sugar – excess glycation

Glycation is simply the attachment of sugar to our protein molecules. 99% of our cellular functions are carried out by proteins, which are absolutely critical to normal life processes within the cell. Proteins are very efficient molecules; they are very slippery long-chain polypeptide molecules that are constantly mingling in the soup inside of the cell (the cytoplasm). As they mingle, they bump into one another, roll around one another, and bounce off of one another – they still get their jobs done, mainly because they are very slippery.

We are all glycating 100% of the time, 24 hours a day, 7 days a week. It's a normal, natural process, yet it's a process detrimental to life. Why? Because since glycation is a passive process of the attachment of sugar to protein molecules, it stands to reason that the higher the blood sugar the more we're going to glycate.

The more sugar that the proteins are exposed to, the more they will attach to. An important thing to understand from this is that when proteins are glycated they become sticky. They start to stick together within the cell and they work much less efficiently. This signals the beginning of cellular dysfunction and inflammation (tissue inflammation). This in turn triggers the process of degenerative disease; basically, poor health (that leads to degenerative conditions) – like atherosclerosis (hardening of the arteries), early heart attacks, strokes and inflammatory diseases. So what this means is that we want to glycate as little as possible.

It is well known that death from old age is becoming rarer and rarer. Nowadays, people are dying of degenerative disease. This is partly based on excess glycation and oxidative stress.

And since glycation is what causes proteins to stick together, which then leads to oxidative stress, we age faster (biologically) when we have high sugar levels.

The other issue is that high sugar levels lead to high insulin levels. As blood sugar goes up, our bodies have to move that sugar from the blood into the cell. That's done by a hormone called insulin.

The Problem with High Sugar – Insulin Resistance

The higher the blood sugar level, the more insulin we have to make, and excess insulin leads to degenerative disease because high insulin levels also cause oxidative stress. If you look at the adult onset diabetic, you will see that they are a model for rapid ageing because they have both high blood sugar and high insulin levels. And long before non-diabetics, they often develop diseases such as atherosclerosis, abnormal cholesterol profile, high blood-pressure, central accumulation of fat (or central obesity), peripheral neuropathy, kidney disease and retinal disease which can lead to blindness.

What has happened with the diabetic is that he/she has developed insulin resistance. Which means that he/she had high sugar and insulin levels for so long, that his/her cells no longer respond to insulin as efficiently as they should. It's a bit like if you had to live next to a noisy train station and you heard the trains day in and day out. Eventually, you would not even hear the trains and your friends would visit and say, "My God, what's that noise?", and you would say, "What noise?" In a similar way, when we have constantly high insulin levels our cells begin to pull in their receptors to insulin, and they stop responding to insulin or they decrease their response to it.

As a result, we develop a problem called insulin resistance, and this happens in both diabetics and non-diabetics. The difference is, in order to develop adult onset diabetes, our insulin resistance increases and increases to the point that our pancreas can't make enough insulin to compensate for it.

As we become more insulin resistant, the pancreas reacts by making more insulin. Higher insulin levels are then necessary to get the cells to pull sugar in from the blood to the cell. As the insulin level continues to get higher and higher, we become even more insulin resistant. So the pancreas compensates by making even more insulin. At some point, the pancreas can't increase insulin production any further. So now you have high sugar, very high insulin, insulin resistance, and the insulin you have isn't enough to bring the sugar from the blood into the cell. The sugar levels go so high that now you're a diabetic.

But it's not only sugar; you're going to find that there are a large number of foods that increase blood sugar rapidly and dramatically that aren't even sweet. It is important to learn what foods those are, because you may not be eating sweets but can still have very high blood sugars by virtue of eating a lot of high glycaemic foods. These will be discussed further in the next chapter.

In conclusion, we can see that whatever affects us physically will affect us mentally, because our body is made up of cells. How we are each affected comes down to our own biochemical individuality. When it comes to how the body uses energy, however, the brain uses proportionally far more – constantly. So anything that affects the way the body uses energy in terms of the body's processes, or if something happens to cause a dysfunction, the brain will be affected. This answers the question of co morbidity: Why is there a high prevalence of, for example, diabetes among people with mental health problems? Why is there a prevalence of heart disease among mental illness sufferers? It's because the body is a whole system: if there is a problem in one area it will impact on another area, either emotionally or in a physical organ itself in terms of deterioration.

I HAVE BEEN asked why I chose to look at nutrition in order to manage and cure my mental illness. It is quite common, when people are experiencing mental illness, that the two things that tend to go out of sync is the person's sleeping and eating pattern. What I realised was that, for example, if I drank tea or coffee, I would become hyper – which meant I couldn't sleep. From that I realised that foods do have an influence; they do impact, and people know this generally because that's why they eat certain foods.

Food influences your mood because it causes the body to release certain hormones, however we have to be careful about what the body is releasing because some of those hormones, in excess or over a prolonged period, can cause illnesses.

What having the proper nutrients inside your body does is to help detoxify the body. Toxins are always circulating through the body, but if you don't consume the necessary nutrients those toxins will accumulate and it's that accumulation that will cause damage.

Having proper amounts of water, vegetables, even vegetable juices, does a lot to help your system in terms of introducing enzymes that break down toxins, reducing their effect and helping them to be flushed out from the body.

3   FOOD AND ITS EFFECTS ON BRAIN FUNCTION

The effects of different foods on our behaviour and cognitive performance have been known for years without needing to be examined closely – caffeine stimulates the brain, when kids have too much sugar they turn 'hyper', and chocolate makes us all feel good. For centuries these experiences have been known and our dietary behaviours reflect this.

Perhaps one of the greatest effects of nutrition on brain function is on our cognition (thinking). The effects of poor diet on sleeping patterns, energy and mood all indirectly affect day to day functioning of the brain at work or school. Cognition is also indirectly affected by the development of other brain functions, which in turn rely on nutrition for their development. For example, nutrition is essential for the development of the sensory systems such as hearing and vision and the integration of these processes – the sensorimotor system. Sensorimotor systems are the coordination between sensory functions and motor (movement) functions. An example of a sensorimotor function would be seeing a ball (sensory) and putting up hands to catch it (motor). These processes mature before cognition as they are essential components needed for learning and memory. Therefore without full and healthy development of these systems, optimal cognitive maturation is not achieved.

Sugar and Altered Glycaemic Load

The brain is an extremely active organ which demands a high percentage of the overall daily energy requirements supplied by food. PET scans and MRIs show which brain areas are utilising the greatest amount of energy by monitoring the glucose consumption. This has enabled scientists to understand the impact of energy on brain development and maturation at different ages.

For infants, 87% of their daily energy intake supplies the brain. In children between the ages of 6-12 years, this reduces to 30 - 45% of their energy. During infancy to early childhood synaptic connectivity is at its greatest rate and therefore glucose utilisation is high. By adulthood, cortical organisation is relatively stable and accordingly the energy demands of the brain decrease to 20-25%. This is still very high considering the brain accounts for only 2% of total body weight.

Our bodies need sugar primarily as a fuel, just like a car needs gas. Blood sugar is usually kept in a healthy range through a set of hormones that send signals in response to our food intake and physical activity. When that control is lost, you end up with lots of sugar in your bloodstream, but can't really use it properly.

Like the flooded carburettor of the older model cars, it is hard to start your engine and you can't get the energy to drive smoothly! With all of that sweet blood, your kidneys cannot cope, and they start to send out the excess sugar in your urine. This condition is called diabetes mellitus, a term of Greek origin meaning a siphoning or 'quick passing through of honey sweet liquid'. Diabetes Mellitus can cause many health complications. For example, it raises the risk of strokes and can lead to blindness and severe foot problems.

So, we all need sugar. Fast-release' sugary foods and drinks, however, cause rapid swings in blood sugar – affecting mood, behaviour and cognition.

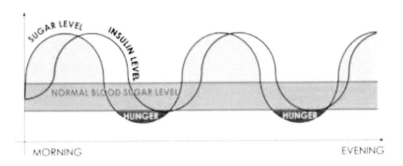

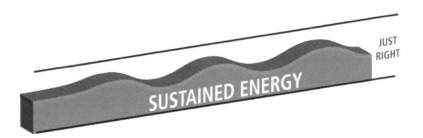

'Slow-release' foods at breakfast help keep blood sugar levels stable – minimising fluctuations in mood, behaviour and cognition.

Addicted To Sugar?

There is evidence that intermittent, excessive sugar intake causes endogenous opioid dependence (Colantuoni, et al., 2002).

In her 1998 book, Kathleen DesMaisons outlined the concept of sugar addiction as a measurable physiological state caused by activation of opioid receptors in the brain, and hypothesised that dependence on sugar followed the same track outlined in the DSM IV for other drugs of abuse.

There is also evidence of opiate-like effects of sugar on gene expression in the reward areas of rat brains (Spangler, et al., 2004).

The human tongue is a highly sensitive area. It permits us to distinguish a wide range of tastes and their nuances. The reason for this sensitivity is the availability of taste buds, which are cells involved in detecting flavours. They are housed inside various projections that stick out of the top surface and sides of the tongue, palate, throat and epiglottis.

In an interview with New Scientist in 2011, Robert Lustig – Professor of Pediatrics at USSF – was asked:

Q: "Why do we consume so much sugar?"

A: "One reason is that it's addictive. The food industry knows that when they add fructose we buy more. That's why it's in everything.

There are five tastes on your tongue:

- Sweet
- Salty
- Sour
- Bitter and
- Umami

Sugar covers up the other four, so you can't taste the negative aspect of foods. You can make a dog poop taste good with enough sugar. In essence, that is what the food industry has done." (Dr. Lustig, 2011).

The Sugar-Craving Cycle

High sugar intake is the enemy of body fat reduction; and the enemy of a healthy, high energy lifestyle. Therefore, it is best to understand what's in the food we're consuming and reduce those that contain more than a few grams of sugar.

Whether it is a can of coke, a scoop of fat-free ice cream, or even a glass of orange juice – all of the ingested sugar quickly rushes into your bloodstream. You typically feel a quick rush of energy. Your body then promptly reacts to this sudden spike in blood sugar by calling on the pancreas to produce additional insulin to remove the excess sugar from your blood, and, for the moment, you have significantly lower blood sugar as a result of the insulin doing its job – resulting in a sense or feeling of needing more fuel, more energy and more calories. As you hit that residual low blood sugar, you begin to crave more of the quick-release, simple sugars. Hence you have just initiated the sugar-craving cycle.

As this downward cycle continues, your pancreas continues to secrete insulin while it simultaneously reduces its production of another hormone called glucagon. Glucagon production, as it relates to improving your body composition, is very important if your fitness goal is to lose excess body fat. Glucagon is the only hormone that allows stored body fat to be released into the bloodstream to be burned by your muscles as energy. And when the pancreas has to elevate its production of insulin while reducing its supply of glucagon, you are basically locking-in your excess body fat. Therefore, too much simple sugar intake dramatically hinders the process of reducing stored body fat.

Think that All Sugars are the Same?

They may all taste sweet to the tongue, but it turns out your body can tell the difference. For example:

Glucose is used by all living cells as a source of energy and is absorbed directly into the bloodstream.

Fructose requires processing by the liver before its energy can be used (technically it is a 'toxin'); no problem if it's consumed via eating fruits and sweet vegetables (the food itself provides the antidote), not healthy if consumed as a 'white powder' e.g. table sugar or high fructose corn syrup (both are approximately 50% glucose and 50% fructose).

The conventional advice to 'Eat less, Exercise more' does not work if eating less still includes eating food high in sugar...because-consuming excess sugar can increase appetite and reduce energy.

In other words, excessive calories from sugar (fructose) affect the balance of key hormones that regulate energy metabolism and appetite. This can in effect lead to insulin resistance, leptin resistance (leptin is a hormone produced by fat cells), increased ghrelin (a gastrointestinal hormone produced by epithelial cells) and so on.

Impact of Foods on Brain Chemistry

Food has a direct impact on the brain and how it functions. Mood, performance, energy, motivation, memory, stress, ageing and concentration can all be affected by nutrients.

The brain and spinal cord comprise the majority of the central nervous system (CNS). Their requirements are much the same as other tissues in the body, yet the CNS needs certain nutrients in order to function optimally. When one or more critical nutrients are lacking from the diet, the result can be neurological disturbances of varying degrees.

For example, neurons of the peripheral nervous system (PNS) can be affected by low levels of vitamin B_6. The effect may be noticeable as neuropathy, or problems with nerve conduction resulting in sensory and motor dysfunction.

Neuropathy can also take place with vitamin B_{12} insufficiency. The National Institutes of Health warns that this can manifest as either numbness or weakness in the legs and arms. More severe vitamin B_{12} deficiency may be observed as bowel and bladder dysfunction and can also lead to impotence in males.

The Problem with Fats

Research shows that unhealthy fats found in dairy products, burgers and milk shakes quickly make their way to the brain, where they shut off the alarm system that tells us when we've had enough to eat. Writing in The Journal of Clinical Investigation, the researchers said that a type of fat called palmitic acid is particularly good at fooling the brain.

In a series of experiments, Dr Clegg showed that saturated fats trick the body into switching off the system that tells us how hungry we are and whether we've eaten enough. The fat makes the brain send out messages telling the body to ignore the information it is getting from the appetite-regulating hormones leptin and insulin.

Dr Clegg, of the University of Texas, said: "Our findings suggest that when you eat something high in fat, your brain gets 'hit' with the fatty acids, and you become resistant to insulin and leptin.

Since you're not being told by the brain to stop eating, you overeat. What we've shown in this study is that someone's entire brain chemistry can change in a very short period of time."

Margarines and commercially baked or fried foods usually contain high levels of hydrogenated and trans fats. These are artificially saturated and 'twisted' fats, which have no known nutritional benefits, but are known to cause many health risks.

Trans fats compete with the essential fatty acids (omega-3 and omega-6) which are needed for brain and body health.

Trans fats: A Real Poison!

In 2009, the World Health Organisation (WHO) declared that trans fats (from hydrogenated vegetable oils) really are toxic, and sensible countries now ban them. Trans fats are artificial 'plastic fats' that raise the risk for:

- Inflammation
- Obesity
- Type 2 diabetes and
- Cardiovascular disease

They are also associated with:

- Depression
- Anxiety
- Memory problems
- Irritability, and
- Aggression

<u>Balancing Omega-3 and Omega-6</u>

A person may not understand the difference between omega-3 and omega-6 fatty acids. They may know that we should increase consumption of the omega-3s, but wonder, "What about omega-6?"

Omega-3 and omega-6 are types of essential fatty acids - meaning we cannot make them on our own and have to obtain them from our diet. Both are polyunsaturated fatty acids that differ from each other in their chemical structure. In modern diets, there are few sources of omega-3 fatty acids, mainly the fat of cold water fish such as salmon, sardines, herring, mackerel, black cod, and bluefish. There are two critical omega-3 fatty acids – Eicosapentaenoic Acid, (EPA) and Docosahexaenoic Acid (DHA) – which the body needs. Vegetarian sources, such as walnuts and flaxseeds, contain a precursor to omega-3 - Alpha-Linolenic Acid (ALA) – that the body must convert to EPA and DHA. EPA and DHA are the building blocks for hormones that control immune function, blood clotting, and cell growth as well as components of cell membranes.

What Are Omega-6s Essential For?

Omega-6 fatty acids are needed for brain function; production and maintenance of bone, skin and hair; regulation of metabolism; and reproductive function. Some omega-6 fatty acids tend to promote inflammation and must be consumed in balanced proportion with omega-3 fatty acids to prevent this.

What are Omega-3s Essential For?

- **Structure of ALL cell membranes:** omega-3 and omega-6 increase membrane fluidity which is essential for optimal cell signalling. 6-10% of the dry mass of the brain should be DHA.   DHA is particularly concentrated in nerve terminals, where chemical signals between cells are exchanged. Concentrations of dopamine, serotonin, noradrenalin, etc. are influenced by omega-3 status. A number of regulatory substances are made from omega-3 and omega-6 Long-Chain Polyunsaturated Fatty Acids (LC-PUFA).

- **Brain development:** omega-3 and omega-6 LC-PUFA make up around 20% of dry brain mass, and affect brain growth and connectivity. For example, the supplementing of infant formula with LC-PUFA (found naturally in breast-milk), can improve visual and cognitive development.

- **Vision:** omega-3 fatty acids from fish oils are absolutely essential to the visual system. 30-50% of the Retina should be made of the omega-3 DHA. At the earliest stages of visual processing, DHA deficiency can reduce retinal signalling by more than a thousand-fold. omega-3 deficiency is associated with poor night vision and other problems with visual, spatial and attentional processing.

Therefore, a healthy balance of omega-6 and omega-3 fatty acids is 2:1 to 4:1 (Sullivan, et al., 2010); (Demar, et al., 2006); (Trevizol, et al., 2011); (Mathieu, Denis, Lavialle, & Vancassel, 2008).

Omega-3 Deficiency In Early Life and Mental Disorders: Evidence For Mechanisms

Omega-3 deficiency during pregnancy has been found to lead to behavioural defects in offspring consistent with anxiety and depression.

Mechanisms now identified include:

- Permanent impairment of endocannabinoid-mediated neural plasticity in hippocampal networks (Lafourcade, et al., 2011).
- Permanent disruption of Brain Derived Neurotrophic Factor (BDNF is a protein that signals brain cells to live and grow), neuropeptide Y-1 and glucocorticoid receptors, and insulin signalling in frontal cortex, hypothalamus and hippocampus. (Bhatia, et al., 2011).
- Short-chain omega-3s (ALAs – as found, for example, in flax oil; rapeseed oil; canola oil;

green leafy vegetables; etc.) are NOT an effective substitute for LC-PUFAs (Brenna, Salem, Sinclair, & Cunnane, 2009).

All of this evidence has implications for non-fish eaters, whose diets provide little or no preformed long-chain omega-3.

Omega-3 and omega-6 fatty acids and their derivatives have very powerful effects on most brain signalling systems. The substances we make from them can profoundly affect hormone balance, blood flow, and immune system function.

Omega-6	Omega-3
From meat, eggs, and dairy-or converted from oils. Gives rise to substances that: • Promote inflammation • Promote blood clotting • Narrow blood vessels	From Fish and seafood-or converted from ALA in green leafy vegetables, flax seed etc. Gives rise to substances that: • Reduce inflammation • Reduce blood clotting • Relax blood vessels

A few simple dietary changes can make a big difference:

- **Eat more:** fish and seafood, green vegetables, nuts and seeds.

- **Eat less:** meat, dairy products and refined vegetable oils.

Evidence from Randomised Controlled Trials (RCTs) demonstrates that:

In relation to dysfunctions of the mind and body, omega-3 from fish and seafood can help to prevent or improve:

- Cardiovascular disease, such as heart disease and stroke.
- Inflammation/Auto-immune disorders, such as Rheumatoid Arthritis.
- Visual problems, related to 'Retinopathy of Prematurity' (ROP, an eye disease that affects prematurely-born babies who have received intensive neonatal care. It is thought to be caused by disorganized growth of retinal blood vessels which may result in scarring and retinal detachment.), diabetes and old age.
- Disorders of behaviour, such as in learning and mood e.g. depression and other mental health problems, ADHD, Dyspraxia, Dyslexia and so on. Depression shows strong associations with diet in both cross-sectional and prospective studies.

High sugar consumption is also associated with depression (over time and across countries), whereas omega-3 fatty acids found in fish and sea foods seem to be a protective factor.

So, unhealthy fat and high sugar consumption are clearly detrimental to not only physical health but also mental well being; they have an indirect effect on cognitive development, function and health. And, as we shall see, they also have an effect on our very behaviour.

WHEN IT COMES to the nervous system and anything that affects the nerves, any fault with that system can cause involuntary movements. At the time when I was experiencing such symptoms I interpreted that as something taking control of me – like a malevolent spirit or something – but now I realise that there was a problem with my nervous system that was causing those behaviours.

Involuntary behaviours such as these are not limited to physical behaviours but also include internal behaviours, like emotions etc.

A person who is not suffering from a mental illness may experience these behaviours during moments of emotional stress – such as throwing objects, which they may find quite startling as they didn't intend to do that! However, when a person is unwell and their system isn't working properly these kinds of things can happen, which all too often leads to these same people ending up on a behavioural disorders unit within a mental health institution.

So, what we do, what we eat, what conditions we're in – in terms of stress etc. – all influence our physical and mental wellbeing. Diet, however, is often overlooked in that equation, but it's a serious thing that people need, at least, to know some basics about in order to truly realise that what we eat affects so much more than our physical health.

The Effect of Nutrition on Genetics and the Brain

Assessments of human nutrition are not complete without consideration of the underlying genetic variability, which may be reflected as differences in nutritional processes such as absorption, metabolism, receptor action, and excretion (Velázquez & Bourges, 1984). Inborn differences in the activity of enzymes and other functional proteins contribute to variations in nutritional requirements and to the differential interaction of certain nutrients with genetically determined biochemical and metabolic factors. There have been numerous studies on the effects of nutrition on genetics and behaviour.

We're learning a lot more about nutrition than before, that were previously only guessed at.

One really exciting area of study is the effect of nutrition on genetics. We're learning that nutrition can control whether genes are operative or non-operative (in other words, whether they are on or off).

We know that the brain uses a tremendous amount of energy. The brain is the only part of the body whose metabolism and function never completely rest.

The brain's metabolism never slows down significantly. Even for people in extremely deep coma, where you have to control respiration, you can only reduce the brain's metabolism by 50%. So, people that are in very deep comas still have quite high metabolism inside their brain.

Because the brain is metabolising these nutrients so rapidly, you produce a lot of free radicals and lipid peroxidation products. That means, you start oxidising the different parts of the brain, which is harmful, and now studies have highlighted that almost all neurological conditions somehow come back to that. Whether it's depression, anxiety, bipolar or schizophrenia; these are all characterised by high free-radical generation, and high process of lipid peroxidation, which begins to destroy the structure of the brain by:

- Destroying its connections

- Destroying the cells, and

- Altering the mitochondria in the DNA.

Unless you replace those damaged parts, brain function begins to fall off, and evidence shows that the effect on the brain is not uniform.

Why? Some parts of the brain are more sensitive than other parts. To give an example of how metabolically active the brain is: The brain consumes about 20% of all the oxygen in the blood, and 25% of all the glucose in the blood, yet it constitutes only 2% of total body weight. So there is an enormous metabolic factory going on in all of these cells inside the brain.

The other thing that's important to note is, just as with all parts of the body, the brain is constantly being replaced. Every component in the brain is replaced – some replacements take years, others decades. Scientific studies are now discovering that some of the most important components, primarily the omega-3 fatty acids like DHA, are replaced extremely rapidly – within about 2 weeks.

What this means is that if you are deficient in DHA omega-3 fatty acids, your brain begins to change its structure very quickly, so that the brain cannot function properly because one of its vital components is missing.

The Effects of Hypoglycaemia

One of the first hints that there might be a connection between what you eat and your behaviour was discovered by Dr. George Gould back in 1910. So we see this is not completely new. Then, in 1935, it was found that hypoglycaemia, low blood sugar, could mimic many of the serious neurological and psychological conditions like anxiety, neurosis, hysteria, neurasthenia (a term first used in 1829 to describe a psychological disorder characterised by chronic fatigue and weakness; a term no longer in scientific use), and even psychosis could be imitated by people becoming hypoglycaemic.

And then, in 1973, Drs. Wendel and Beebe found that there was a 74% incidence of hypoglycaemia in people who had schizophrenia, the type of schizophrenia associated with anxiety. In other words, in very hyperactive schizophrenics, close to three quarters of them were hypoglycaemic.

Other studies have revealed a close correlation between alcohol abuse, hypoglycaemia and criminal behaviour. In a study it was found that 97% of alcoholics were hypoglycaemic compared to 18% for the controls (Poulos, Stoddard, & Carron, 1976). The reason the alcoholic continues to drink alcohol is because the alcohol is a source of tremendous energy. So when their blood sugar falls and they drink the alcohol they feel better, and when their blood sugar falls again, they drink more alcohol. It becomes an unending cycle.

What the studies also revealed is that if the hypoglycaemia was treated, 71% of alcoholics became sober. Meanwhile, Alcoholics Anonymous' best rate was 25%. So correcting one condition corrected another.

In the United States, FBI statistics show that most of the violent crimes are connected to alcohol. For example, most car accidents and road rage incidences are connected to alcohol. This is because the alcohol is producing the same effect that sugar produces. The most aggressive effect of this is seen in people who have abnormalities of the temporal lobe of the brain. The temporal lobe is not just for memory, but it's the elaboration centre for your emotions – particularly things like anger. It connects to the Amygdala Nucleus in the brain, which controls anger, and it's been found that if a person with temporal lobe dysfunction becomes hypoglycaemic they can become enraged. These are some of the people that have been found to exhibit road rage. They are the people who in a moment of anger could stomp somebody to death, or pick up a knife and stab somebody to death, seemingly out of the blue, for things that are seen as minor to most of us and that most of us would just shrug off.

The reason for this is because the hypoglycaemia triggers their temporal lobe (specifically their anger centre, in their temporal lobe), which causes them to lose all control. This is referred to by a term known as Episodic Dyscontrol Syndrome (EDS).

Interestingly, it is said that if an electrode was put on the temporal lobe of the brain, which stimulated that centre, you would attack whoever was closest to you and you'd try to kill them, you would not be able to stop yourself.

<u>Study On the Influence of Hypoglycaemia on Behaviour</u>

In a Finnish study of violent offenders in prison, it was found that in excessively violent offenders – the ones who would attack you out of the blue and beat you senseless or stomp you to death – their blood sugar fell suddenly and rose very quickly. In other words, those whose blood sugar would fall and then come back up quickly were found to be the ones who exhibited most violence. It was found that the anti-social offender (that is the person who steals and shoplifts, but is not necessarily violent), his blood sugar would also fall but then it would be slow to rise in coming back up (Virkkunen, 1983).

As we know, the changes in blood sugar can produce dramatic alterations in brain function, this is said to influence these anti-social behaviours.

In fact, there were even cases in which it was found that people would tend toward kleptomania because of a high sugar intake.

Further studies are showing a strong connection between sugar metabolism, carbohydrate metabolism in the brain and various psychological conditions. For example, psychosis has been associated with glucose metabolism impairment (Lasevoli, et al., 2012).

The Problem with Hypoglycaemia

1. When sugar is in excess it produces an excess release of insulin.

2. When excessive insulin is released you get hypoglycaemia (that is, the sugar level falls).

When the blood sugar level falls, a number of things happen. Your body tries to get that blood sugar back up because it needs the sugar for its energy metabolism. So it stimulates the adrenal gland to release two hormones: epinephrine and norepinephrine. These are the hormones that make you jittery and nervous when your blood sugar falls, and they stimulate the brain to increase activity. Also, when the brain becomes hypoglycaemic it releases one of its neurotransmitters called glutamate. Glutamate is the primary neurotransmitter for excitability; it is the primary thing that switches the brain's activity into a high gear. So both of these (the norepinephrine and epinephrine) together with glutamate are producing a state of hyperactivity.

Sugar and Processed Foods

Multiple large, controlled studies have shown that the amount of sugar in your diet has a direct influence in terms of criminal behaviour, and drives the inclination towards violent acts and towards anti-social behaviour. This is a cause for a great concern, as the majority of us are consuming more sugars than ever.

57% of this sugar comes from processed foods, and it's not always about putting a spoon of sugar in your coffee, often it's hidden in your food – particularly processed foods. One of the leading sources of sugar in our diets is soft drinks – fruit juices, cokes, etc. 43% of all sugars are coming from these sources, and if you go anywhere where there are a lot of young people, you'll often see that they are drinking these types of high sugar, caffeinated beverages.

People say, "It's mostly young people," and they may be right, because if you look at adverts for Coca Cola and Pepsi, for example, they're mostly targeted at the younger generation. And what do mothers do when their babies get old enough to be weaned? They often give their toddler those little cartons of fruit juice drink. Just one of those cartons can contain as much as 35 grams of sugar. These carton orange and berry juices drinks are extremely high in sugar. So children get started early on sugars and get used to high sugar intake.

It's not surprising then, that when it comes to teenagers, research has revealed that they are drinking an equivalent of up to 54 teaspoons of sugar a day just from the consumption of soft drinks. Most nutritionists would limit the sugar intake to around 10 teaspoons per day. The real consumption of sugars may be even double or triple the amount stated, due to the fact that many soft drinks are available in large sized bottles.

According to a report in the Guardian in February 2013, "Sugar is behind the global explosion in type 2 diabetes. Researchers say the link between sugar consumption and diabetes is independent from obesity; it plays a uniquely damaging role in causing a disease that experts fear could overwhelm the NHS." Researchers were led by Sanjay Basu, an assistant professor at Stanford University school of medicine, who examined the availability of sugar and diabetes rates from 175 countries worldwide over the last decade.

Metabolically, we know that when you consume a lot of sugar, it dramatically increases free-radical generation in your brain. This produces a cross-linking of the proteins in all your cells that significantly increases the damaging effects of these free radicals.

What this means is that over time, the sugar moieties (sugar components of DNA) bound to the glycated proteins are chemically modified to become Advanced Glycation Endproducts (AGEs), forming covalent 'cross-links' with adjacent protein strands. This cross-linking (between DNA and protein) stiffens tissues which were formerly flexible or elastic. Cross-linking of this kind causes damage to the DNA molecule and must be repaired before DNA can replicate and function properly again.

The bottom line is, it makes every cell in your body age much faster, particularly brain cells. To illustrate, what studies are highlighting is that people who consume a lot of calories, particularly in refined sugar, their incidence of Alzheimer's Disease is about six times higher than everybody else's.

<u>Is Refined Sugar Toxic?</u>

In 1957, Dr. William Coda Martin tried to answer the question: When is a food a food and when is it a poison? His working definition of 'poison' was: "Medically: Any substance applied to the body, ingested or developed within the body, which causes or may cause disease. Physically: Any substance which inhibits the activity of a catalyst, which is a minor substance, chemical or enzyme that activates a reaction." The dictionary gives an even broader definition for 'poison': 'to exert a harmful influence on, or to pervert'.

Dr. Martin classified refined sugar as a poison because it has been depleted of its life forces, vitamins and minerals. "What is left consists of pure, refined carbohydrates. The body cannot utilise this refined starch and carbohydrate unless the depleted proteins, vitamins and minerals are present. Nature supplies these elements in each plant in quantities sufficient to metabolise the carbohydrate in that particular plant. There is no excess for other added carbohydrates. Incomplete carbohydrate metabolism results in the formation of 'toxic metabolite', such as pyruvic acid, and abnormal sugars containing five carbon atoms. Pyruvic acid accumulates in the brain and nervous system, and the abnormal sugars in the red blood cells. These toxic metabolites interfere with the respiration of the cells. They cannot get sufficient oxygen to survive and function normally. In time, some of the cells die. This interferes with the function of a part of the body and is the beginning of degenerative disease."

So, refined sugar is harmful when ingested by humans because it provides that which nutritionists describe as "empty" or "naked" calories. It lacks the natural minerals which are present in the sugar beet or cane.

The Problem with Refined Sugar

Refined sugar is, in fact, a nutrient siphon, draining and leaching the body of precious vitamins and minerals through the demand that its digestion, detoxification and elimination makes upon our entire system. Because balance is so essential, our bodies have many ways to work against the sudden shock of a heavy intake of sugar. Minerals such as sodium (from salt), potassium and magnesium (from vegetables), and calcium (from the bones) are mobilised and used in chemical transformation. Neutral acids are produced in an attempt to return the acid-alkaline balance factor of the blood to a more normal state.

Therefore, refined sugars taken every day, produce a continuously over-acid condition, and more and more minerals are required from deep in the body in the attempt to rectify the imbalance.

Finally, in order to protect the blood, so much calcium is taken from the bones and teeth that decay and general weakening begin. Excess sugar eventually affects every organ in the body. Initially, it is stored in the liver in the form of glucose (glycogen). Since the liver's capacity is limited, a daily intake of refined sugar (above the required amount of natural sugar) soon makes the liver expand like a balloon. When the liver is filled to its maximum capacity, the excess glycogen is returned to the blood in the form of fatty acids. These are taken to every part of the body and stored in the most inactive areas such as the belly, the buttocks, the breasts and the thighs.

When these comparatively harmless places are completely filled, fatty acids are then distributed among active organs, such as the heart and kidneys. These begin to slow down; finally their tissues degenerate and turn to fat.

The whole body is affected by their reduced ability, and abnormal blood pressure is created. The parasympathetic nervous system is affected, and organs governed by it, such as the small brain, become inactive or paralysed (normal brain function is rarely thought of as being as biologic as digestion). The circulatory and lymphatic systems are invaded, and the quality of the red corpuscles starts to change. An overabundance of white cells occurs, and the creation of tissue becomes slower. Our body's tolerance and immunising power becomes more limited, so we cannot respond properly to extreme attacks, whether they be cold, heat, mosquitoes or microbes.

As can be seen, excessive sugar has a strong mal-effect on both the body and the functioning of the brain. The key to orderly brain function is glutamic acid, a vital compound found in many vegetables. The B vitamins play a major role in dividing glutamic acid into antagonistic-complementary compounds which produce a 'proceed' or 'control' response in the brain. B vitamins are also manufactured by symbiotic bacteria which live in our intestines. When refined sugar is taken daily, these bacteria wither and die, and our stock of B vitamins gets very low.

A Provocative Research on the Relationship between Diet and Mental Illness

Noted British psychiatric researcher Malcolm Peet has conducted a provocative cross-cultural analysis of the relationship between diet and mental illness. His primary finding may surprise you: a strong link between high sugar consumption and the risk of both depression and schizophrenia.

In fact, there are two potential mechanisms through which refined sugar intake could exert a toxic effect on mental health.

First, sugar actually suppresses activity of a key protein in the brain called BDNF, which you may remember from the previous chapter. This protein promotes the health and maintenance of neurons in the brain, and it plays a vital role in memory function by triggering the growth of new connections between neurons. BDNF levels are critically low in both depression and Schizophrenia, which explains why both syndromes often lead to shrinkage of key brain regions over time (yes, chronic depression actually leads to brain damage).

Second, high sugar consumption triggers a cascade of chemical reactions in the body that promote chronic inflammation. Now, under certain circumstances (like when your body needs to heal an insect bite), a little inflammation can be a good thing, since it can increase immune activity and blood flow to a wound, but in the long term inflammation is a big problem. It disrupts the normal functioning of the immune system, and wreaks havoc on the brain.

Inflammation is associated with an increased risk of heart disease, diabetes, arthritis, and even some forms of cancer. It's also linked to a greater risk of depression and schizophrenia, and, again, eating refined sugar triggers inflammation.

The dietary predictors of outcome in schizophrenia and prevalence of depression are similar to those that predict illnesses such as coronary heart disease and diabetes, which are more common in people with mental health problems and in which nutritional approaches are widely recommended. Dietary intervention studies are now indicated in schizophrenia and depression.

This new research is shedding much needed light on the reality that diet does indeed play a role in the incidence of mental illness.

Dr. Ilardi, associate professor of psychology at the University of Kansas, stated that he encouraged depressed patients to remove refined sugar and refined foods from their diets. Patients who were willing to comply with these recommendations reported significant improvements in mental clarity, mood and energy. Research and patient experiences indicate that a diet high in whole grains and low in refined foods and sugars can provide significant improvement in mental health, clarity and reduced risk of mental illness.

A Relationship between Crime and Nutritional Status?

In the United States, a study of prison systems in five different states looked at adult criminal offenders. The studies looked for deficiencies in a lot of different nutrients but mainly magnesium, zinc, folate and vitamin B_6.

What they found in all five states was that violent offenders had the most deficiencies of all the prisoners; the more violent, the more nutritional deficiencies were found.

Another study carried out by the Alabama prison service demonstrated that when the diet of criminals was changed, there was a 42% reduction in criminal events, and there was a 61% reduction in anti-social behaviour within one year. This is just another of the many studies showing the profound effect of diet.

So is the problem just hypoglycaemia?

A study at an Oklahoma children's centre did a similar nutritional study, and they found there was a 43% reduction in serious crime when they changed the diet. This came about because they got rid of the high fat, high sugar diet and junk foods that the child offenders were on. When the researchers wanted to see whether there was any objective evidence of change in brain function, they looked at EEGs in the brain function of the offenders. What they found is that there were about 14 different abnormalities in their EEGs.

When they switched their diet it went from 14 to 2 abnormalities. So the EEGs improved considerably and one child went from 6 to 0 abnormalities after being given a simple vitamin supplement.

The researchers also found that even marginal deficiencies in nutrition could cause criminal behaviour to surface in these susceptible individuals.

Selenium

Several of these researches identified selenium (an essential trace mineral found in foods such as brazil nuts, sunflower seeds, bran, liver and fish) as one of the nutritional elements involved in brain function. There are a number of studies on selenium and brain function. Some researchers have commented, "Before, we thought selenium mainly had to do with things like anti-oxidant activity. We thought it was for the health of the liver and heart. Now, we understand that actually it has things to do with the functioning of the brain itself, particularly in terms of behaviour."

Studies have found that deficiencies in selenium are commonly associated with depression and periods of confusion and that when you elevate the selenium intake, there is a significant improvement in people's mood (Schweizer, Bräuer, Köhrle, Nitsch, & Savaskan, 2004).

More recent studies have shown that selenium does indeed play a major role in how the brain functions. So deficiency is very detrimental to the brain.

Food Sensitivities and Behaviour

A study reported in the Lancet suggests that food sensitivities may be quite common among behaviourally-disturbed children. 81 out of a group of 140 children with behaviour disorders (almost two-thirds) experienced significant improvement following the elimination of certain foods along with food additives. When they were challenged with the specific foods which had been eliminated, their behaviour problems returned. Moreover, 75% of these children reacted to a double-blind challenge with salicylates (a type of chemical that occurs naturally in plants and found in many fruits, herbs and vegetables) but not to placebo (Swain, Soutter, Loblay, & Truswell, 1985).

The following case study, reported in Psychology Today, illustrates how food sensitivities may affect aggressive behaviour:

When he was five years and one month old, G.L. was seen because of uncontrollable temper tantrums. He was believed aphasic because of poor speech development, and was too uncomfortable to do initial IQ testing. The EEG showed 14-per-second spikes; large amounts of sharp activity in the motor leads; temporal single, polyphasic sharp waves; and a long run of sharp waves in the right temporal area. Allergy tests revealed strong reactions to milk, chocolate and yeast.

He was placed on a diet free of milk, chocolate, and cola drinks. Seven and one half months later, his EEG was normal. Six months after the repeat EEG, he was learning better and his behaviour was much improved. He was challenged again with the suspected foods for one week, during which time his behaviour again became uncontrollable.

The EEG now showed two-and-one-half to six-per-second activity on the right, greater in the mid-temporal and parietal leads, accentuated by drowsiness. Light cerebral dysfunction was diagnosed (Moyer, 1975).

Adults may also display overaggressive behaviours due to food sensitivities. For example, Mackarness has written of a woman who had been hospitalised thirteen times for violent behaviour and depression; after common foods were eliminated from her diet, she no longer became violent or depressed. Instead she felt fine and obtained a regular job (MacKarness, 1976).

While the research literature suggests that any commonly ingested food or food additive may be responsible for provoking pathological psychological and behavioural reactions, milk may be a special case. Schauss and Simonsen found that chronic juvenile delinquents consumed much more milk than matched controls without a history of delinquency. The male offenders consumed an average of a gallon of milk daily compared to a little less than a quart a day for the controls, and the females showed similar differences (Schauss & Simonsen, 1979).

Schauss believes that overconsumption of milk causes antisocial behaviour. He has reported that, when several Michigan detention centres reduced their inmates' milk consumption, the incidence of antisocial behaviour declined; when they permitted milk consumption to increase again, antisocial behaviour also increased (Schauss, Nutrition and antisocial behaviour, 1984).

Glucose can covalently bind to DNA by a non-enzymatic process as a result of glycation. Glycation of DNA is of special interest due to its possible influence on the functionality of DNA (cross-linking) and overall effect on gene expression (epigenetics).

In the following chapter we'll be taking a look at epigenetics and its role in the expression of genes, thereby determining our path towards health or disease.

ONE OF THE proofs for nutritional therapy is obviously within my own self: when I was in hospital I was told I would never be well without medication, however I've successfully used nutrition to aid my recovery. In contrast to that is what has happened to both my mum and brother. So, that's on a personal level – I can see that they're still dependent on medication and will probably remain so.

But there's also a lot of research to support nutrition as mental health therapy. In particular epigenetics. Epigenetics is about gene expression which, as opposed to genes which are fixed, can change throughout a person's lifetime. What you eat and the lifestyle you adopt can actually change the genetic expression of what happens to you in terms of health or illness, and these changes can be passed on to the next generation.

The body needs certain nutrients that medication can't provide, so as the body is going through the normal stresses of day to day living, and toxins are building up in the body, the body – being nutrient deficient – cannot get rid of them. These toxins in turn affect the epigenetic element of one's genes, switching genes off and on for certain physical and mental disorders. The potential for these negative gene expressions to be passed on to our children is very significant here, showing that a healthy diet and lifestyle is not just for our own benefit.

5 EPIGENETICS: MENTAL HEALTH AND NUTRIENT THERAPY

It is clear that the quality and quantity of food we eat shapes the body, but how permanent is the impact on us as a whole in terms of our genes?

New landmark research indicates that you can greatly influence what genes are switched on or off, through diet and enzyme activity. Food doesn't just fill us up, it affects our genes.

<u>The Expression of Genes Can Be Changed!</u>

Scientists are now saying over 95% of human disease is epigenetically determined. In other words, you can't change your genes but you can change the way your genes are expressed.

The modulation of epigenetic status has been strongly implicated in the etiology of disease, and it is modifiable by diet and lifestyle.

Historically, it was thought that disease was caused through direct mutation of the genome. However, there are very few diseases that have been shown to be associated with mutation, meaning that the vast majority of diseases must be caused by other alterations.

Environmental conditions can cause disease through changing of individual cell types or the individual themselves, which would later cause disease. This means that epigenetics provides the missing link on how the environment can change the cell without causing mutation to induce disease. And nutrition is a major environmental factor that affects the healthy organism.

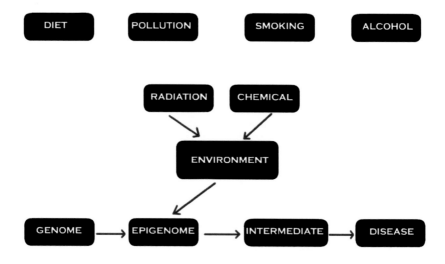

Unlike the genome, the epigenome is much more flexible and dynamic. Meaning that it changes over time in response to a number of different environmental factors. These include diet, pollution, lifestyle factors such as smoking, alcohol and stress, radiation and chemical exposure. This is linked to disease, as altering the epigenome will alter whether genes are active or inactive in such a way that the activity could be on when they should be off, or off when they should be on – potentially causing disease, as gene expression is usually a tightly controlled process. Findings have also clearly shown that epigenetic changes can also be passed on to subsequent generations.

So, What Is Epigenetics?

Epigenetics (which literally means 'in addition to changes in genetic sequence') is the study of gene expression. It's how your genes turn on and off-its gene signalling.

What scientists have long known is that your genes stay the same (they're passed down from your parents); although there may be mutations here and there, they're not really going to affect your actual gene structure.

On the other hand, your gene expression is going to change dramatically over your lifespan, and is controlled by your epigenetics. What scientists have now found is that there are 'markers' on the outside of your genes (a bit like a light switch) that attach to DNA telling a cell to either use or ignore a particular gene. In other words, they turn your genes on, off, up slightly or down slightly. These epigenetic changes are what are believed to make the biggest impact on your health.

For example: In a study, scientists found that when they gave Agouti mice certain toxins, it turned on their epigenetic switch for a particular one of their genes: an obesity gene. The mice ate a lot of food, gained weight rapidly, got tired and had a lot of fatigue. The mice also rapidly developed diabetes and heart disease, and often cancer as well. These changes were caused by the epigenetic switches and these epigenetic switches were changed by their diet.

So the more toxins we consume – such as those found in fast foods and junk foods – the more we are going to turn the bad genes on and the good genes off. It's a gradual process, so the longer we consume a poor diet, the more epigenetic switches are turned the bad way. Conversely, the longer we consume a healthy diet the more our epigenetic switches are going to turn the good way. It's also important to note that the process of epigenetic marking is fundamental to homeostasis and healthy functioning of cells.

Epigenetic Switches can be Passed Down from One Generation to the Next

What's interesting about the mice study is that scientists found that these epigenetic switches could be passed down from one generation to the next generation. What this means is that the choices we make today about what we eat and how healthy we want our lifestyle to be will be passed on to our children.

In the mice study, scientists found that when epigenetic switches for obesity were turned on, the mice gave birth to obese offspring. What this demonstrated was that some epigenetic switches were passed down.

Something else the scientists learnt was that when the obese mice were pregnant and fed with a dose of anti-oxidants (phytonutrients from fruits, vegetables, berries etc.), it turned the obesity gene off for the offspring and the pregnant mice gave birth to normal, healthy young, even though the mother still suffered from obesity, was sick and eventually died.

The most common epigenetic mark is a methyl group. When these groups fasten to DNA through a process called methylation they block the attachment of proteins which normally turn the genes on. As a result, the gene is turned off.

What We Eat Has the Ability to Impact Our Genetic Expression via Methylation

Methylation is a key process that is essential for almost all body processes, and it occurs billions of times every second. If you look at the science of epigenetics for various disorders, methylation appears to be the most powerful factor.

Methylation is a chemical process that occurs in every cell of the body. It is essential for many critical functions such as DNA and RNA synthesis and expression, glutathione conjugation and synthesis, and synthesis of neurotransmitters such as dopamine, serotonin and GABA. Proper methylation is also essential for immune regulation, including viral inhibition.

Scientists have witnessed epigenetic inheritance, the observation that offspring may inherit altered traits due to their parents' past experiences. For example, historical incidences of famine (Study: Amsterdam Netherlands History, 1944-45) have resulted in health effects on the children and grandchildren of individuals who had restricted diets, possibly because of inheritance of altered epigenetic marks caused by a restricted diet.

Nutritional Therapy Protocols for Mental and Behavioural Disorders

Epigenetic Study by Dr. William J. Walsh Ph.D - Research Institute, Naperville, IL

"I'm so excited about epigenetics," Dr. Walsh tells the Irish Medical Times, "this is the most exciting thing that has happened in 40 years. It appears many of the diseases we thought were genetic are actually epigenetic," he said. "Epigenetics has the advantage that it can lead to therapies that can reverse what genes are doing."

Epigenetics "provides a roadmap to more effective therapies for mental and behavioural disorders, because the primary method for helping these kinds of problems over the last 30 to 40 years has been psychiatric medications."

Dr. Walsh continued by saying, "I think our next step will be to use our knowledge of molecular biology and brain chemistry to find ways to directly correct neurotransmitter and receptor problems. We're getting closer to understanding exactly what goes wrong and reversing how this occurs."

Have Doctors Really Forgotten What They Learnt in Medical School?

"There's a belief that you need a powerful drug to treat a problem like schizophrenia or bipolar disorder, but I think a lot of doctors have forgotten what they learnt in medical school: Where do neurotransmitters come from? What factors affect neurotransmitter uptake and the process of synapse?"

Nutrient therapy can be a key to treating mental and behavioural disorders (according to Dr. Walsh). "When you dig into the molecular biology of this, you find nutrient factors are extremely important. If a person had a genetic disorder that caused them to be very deficient in vitamin B_6, well, this is the major core factor in the production of serotonin. So, if a person has a major B_6 deficiency, you can be sure they'll be low in serotonin and will suffer from depression, or at least have a tendency for it."

So what's the answer? "The solution could be to prescribe fluoxetine, or selective serotonin reuptake inhibitor medication to help with side-effects, but it seems a lot more scientific, if a person is depressed, to simply normalize their B_6 levels. If you do a complete metabolic analysis of any human, you'll find they'll probably be low in five or six important nutrient factors because of genetics and epigenetics. If you could identify these, the person may benefit from many times the RDA of those nutrients, because they're fighting genetics." Dr. Walsh explained. Dr. Walsh continued by explaining that the treatment weapons he uses are amino acids, fatty acids, and vitamins and minerals, focusing on nutrients that have a powerful impact on the synthesis of neurotransmitters or what happens when an electrical impulse crosses the synapse.

Many mental disorders have perplexed scientists for years, because illnesses like depression run in families.

"The problem is these illnesses violate the classic laws of genetics," says Dr. Walsh. "I think we now have the answers because it's really epigenetics, not genetics. The conditions don't involve changes in the DNA, but the changes involved are alterations or modifications – errors, you might say – in gene expression."

Is There Really No Way to Avoid Heritable Mental Illnesses?

There is increasing evidence that epigenetic mechanisms play a major role in the pathogenesis of psychiatric disorders (Peedicayil, 2007).

Until recently, all heritable mental illnesses were presumed to have an unavoidable genetic component. That is, people have been misled to believe that their biological and psychological fate has already been predetermined and is locked in by gene mutations.

Many features of psychiatric diseases are consistent with an epigenetic dysregulation such as discordance of monozygotic twins, late age of onset, parent-of-origin and sex effects, and fluctuating disease course. (Ptak & Petronis, 2010).

Dr. Walsh asks, "If these mental disturbances are inevitable, why don't identical twins follow a Mendelian pattern on inheritance?"

One study in particular was conducted on 22 pairs of identical twins. Identical twins have identical DNA. However one twin among each pair expressed bipolar or schizophrenia, and the other did not. Researchers investigated why this was the case despite having identical DNA. In the mentally ill twin, researchers found significant changes in how certain genes were methylated. In some cases, there was significant over and under methylation of certain genes that were present, due to epigenetic alterations. This meant that some type of environmental influence was responsible for causing the mental illness in the identical twin. Environment can be anything from diet, nutrient deficiencies and toxicity, to the impact of physical trauma and stress on how the genes are expressed. This means that genes do not rule you as much as your diet, lifestyle, toxicity-related factors and stress may rule how your genes express mental illness (as well as huge groups of other disease processes).

Dr. Walsh Case Study Examples

In his book, Dr. Walsh presents the case of a 21 year old male diagnosed with paranoid schizophrenia, the same condition that had affected his mother. This patient arrived for his first evaluation wearing a metal helmet and had chains wrapped around his neck, which he said were necessary to keep him from floating up into outer space. He also believed his parents were aliens from outer space.

His biochemical imbalances were treated with a regimen of vitamins and minerals. He wasn't always compliant in taking the vitamin and mineral supplements, but after six months significant improvement was reported. After several years of wellness, a gap in his nutritional regimen resulted in a return of his delusions. He resumed his nutritional regimen and returned to wellness.

Another case presented by Dr. Walsh involved a 22 year old student with schizophrenia. He told friends that Russians agents were trying to kill him, and would sit for hours with a blank expression. Once diagnosed, he was medicated with mind-altering drugs (Zyprexa, Depakote and Zoloft) which resulted in improvement, but he couldn't hold a job or resume studies. A nutritional regimen did not produce any change for six weeks, followed by gradual improvement. After a year of nutrient therapy a near-complete recovery was reported and he was weaned away from drugs.

Dr Walsh has demonstrated that advanced nutrient therapy can be effective by:

- Normalising the synthesis of our brain chemicals,

- Adjusting activity at brain cell receptors by alteration of gene expression, and

- Defending against oxidative stress.

In his book 'Nutrient Power' Dr. Walsh states that epigenetics has identified several nutrient factors that have a powerful impact on transporters at neurotransmitter synapses, including methionine, SAMe, folic acid, niacinamide, and zinc. In addition, epigenetics has identified several other nutrients with potential for improving brain functioning. Since nutrient therapy involves normalising of brain chemistry, this approach has the great advantage of minimal adverse side-effects. In effect, methionine and SAMe are natural serotonin reuptake inhibitors, while folic acid increases genetic expression of transporters, causing reduced activity of dopamine and serotonin. Folate and methyl produce opposite effects on neurotransmission; Folic is a serotonin reuptake enhancer, whereas methionine and SAMe are serotonin reuptake inhibitors.

The new science of epigenetics rewrites the rules of disease, heredity and identity. "We have shown, in a general sense, how nutrients can often accomplish what drugs hope to achieve, but in a more natural manner that is less prone to adverse side-effects," says Dr. Walsh.

I CAME ACROSS some very interesting books by people who were, so called, 'thinking outside the box' in terms of mental health. Carl Pfeiffer was one of them; he had done a lot of research on orthomolecular nutrition – the study of preventing and curing disease with nutrition. From there I learned some things regarding the role of essential nutrients and the use of vitamins to help with certain types of mental illness.

Vitamin supplements have helped me, especially b-complex supplements. What I've found is that when I go without b-complex for a while I become tearful and begin to get depressed. I went through a phase where I didn't have it for a while, because it was quite expensive, but I found that I was becoming tearful. I went to my doctor and tried to explain that I needed b-complex, but she apologised and said she could not prescribe it. She offered me antidepressants and also therapy – if I wanted to go for that.

I took the prescription from her but I didn't process it because it wasn't what I wanted. I went back to buying the vitamin b-complex and I was fine again.

We all need a balanced diet, one that's going to balance us as individuals. This means paying attention to those nutrients that the body cannot make itself, those essential nutrients that must be included in our diets.

Oxidative Stress

Cell health equals overall health.

All disease originates at the cellular level and not at the organ or system level.   Healthy cells create healthy tissues.

So what constitutes a healthy cell? What we eat, drink, breathe and bathe in will either nourish the 75 trillion cells in our bodies with oxygen, water, vitamins, minerals and phytonutrients, essential fatty acids, glucose and amino acids, or contaminate cells by the slow poisoning of the blood stream. Brain cells are more vulnerable than other cells to oxidative damage because the brain consumes about 20% of the body's total oxygen although it constitutes less than 2% of total body weight.

The significance of oxidative damage as a component of many disease processes in the central nervous system is being increasingly recognised. Oxidative stress has been found in neurological disorders such as Parkinson's disease and Alzheimer's disease, and it was identified in mental illnesses such as bipolar disorder and schizophrenia.

Oxidative stress is defined as a disturbance in the balance between the production of reactive oxygen species, in other words free-radicals and antioxidant defences. It has been implicated in the development of morbid conditions and mechanisms underlying psychiatric disorders. For example, there is evidence to support the conclusion that oxidative stress mechanisms are involved in schizophrenia.

Studies have shown that intake of antioxidant nutrients can counteract the negative inflammatory results related to mental disorders. Schizophrenics who are given fatty acids and antioxidants showed significant improvements in psychological tests as well as quality of life (Arvindakshan, Ghate, Ranjekar, Evans, & Mahadik, 2003).

<u>Antioxidants</u>

The benefits of fruits and vegetables may be due, in part, to antioxidants and other micronutrients. Oxidant by-products of normal energy metabolism – superoxide, hydrogen, peroxide and hydroxyl radical – are the same mutagens produced by radiation.

Ingesting inadequate amounts of dietary antioxidants – such as vitamin C and E – mimics radiation exposure. Oxidative damage to DNA and other macromolecules appears to have a major role in ageing and degenerative diseases associated with ageing.

Oxidative Stress and Telomeres

"We age because our cells divide and our telomeres get shorter."
(Dr. Andrews, 2011)

Dr. William H. Andrews, Ph.D, a world leading researcher on telomeres, is also a principle discoverer of RNA and protein components of human telomeres.

At this point you may be asking: What are telomeres?

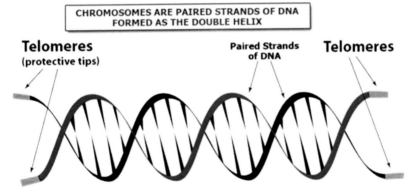

CHROMOSOMES ARE PAIRED STRANDS OF DNA
FORMED AS THE DOUBLE HELIX

Telomeres
(protective tips)

Paired Strands
of DNA

Telomeres

Every cell contains a nucleus with genes and chromosomes. The chromosomes are made up of DNA molecules that are one hundred base pairs long, coiled up. There are long repetitive sequences of DNA at the end of each pair of chromosomes. These sequences are called telomeres. Telomeres act like the tips on the end of shoelaces. These string-like chromosomes have caps (telomeres) on their tips, so that the strands don't unravel.

<u>Why Are Telomeres Important?</u>

Each time our cells divide, these chromosomes divide as well. The problem is that these little tips of telomere get shorter each time the cell divides.

When the cell divides, the genetic material inside that cell needs to be copied. This is called DNA replication. During this process enzymes that replicate a strand of DNA are unable to continue replicating all the way to the end, which causes loss of some DNA. And the ends, if you remember, are where the telomeres are. As telomeres get shorter, the general effects of ageing are initiated:

- Loss of muscle
- Failing memory
- Poor eyesight
- Lack of energy and
- Slower recovery from exercise

The bottom line is this, when cells divide, telomeres shorten and bad things happen when telomeres get short.

However, all is not lost. Research has shown that there are some things that can be done such as lifestyle changes. Specifically: decreasing toxins in our body, addressing obesity, improving our nutrition, reducing physical and mental oxidative stress – all of which are key to slowing down the ageing process.

Research completed by Dr. Williams and his team in 1997 established that humans also have an enzyme called telomerase that can lengthen telomeres. This research was so significant, that in 2009 it was awarded the Nobel Prize in Physiology or Medicine.

Researchers are now correlating telomere life, not just with age, but with general health as well.

You may be wondering 'how is this relevant to mental health'?

What is one substance that we produce in ourselves that is absolutely critical for the preservation of telomere length?

GLUTATHIONE: The most important antioxidant available to the immune system. It is also important in controlling the signs of ageing and for overall physical and mental health. Glutathione is beneficial in promoting sleep and improving mental disorders.

Studies show a direct correlation with schizophrenia and decreased glutathione levels. Studies also show that glutathione can slow down and lessen the side-effects of drugs given to manage schizophrenia.

Your body makes glutathione but many factors contribute to its depletion. Including foods that are precursors to glutathione in your diet is a better way to increase levels of the antioxidant than taking supplements.

Micronutrients from food can help maintain the oxygen balance in your brain. They can help beneficial oxygen reach your brain as well as combat the highly-reactive forms of oxygen called free radicals. Strong evidence suggests that oxygen free radicals may play an important role in the pathophysiology of major mental illnesses such as schizophrenia (Zhang, Zhao, He, & Wan, 2010).

If free radicals get out of control, cells will be damaged faster than they can be repaired. Like a biological form of rust, a lifetime of oxidative insult can lead to diminished brain function.

At the molecular level, biochemistry becomes physics. The atoms in a chemical bond share a pair of electrons that create a magnetic attraction. These atomic bonds are constantly breaking and reforming. When a bond breaks, each atom reclaims its electron and briefly becomes a free radical, an unstable molecule that immediately seeks to pair up with another atomic partner. Antioxidants (anti-oxygen) are your first line of defence against free radicals. Free radicals are a normal part of metabolism and play a vital role in many biochemical processes, but they must be kept under control (The Franklin Institute, 2004).

Antioxidants work in your body to counteract the effects of free radicals, which cause cellular damage that results in a variety of health conditions. In a sense, antioxidants sacrifice themselves to preserve your body parts. They readily donate their electrons to prevent free radicals from stealing electrons out of membrane fatty acids, mitochondria, DNA, and elsewhere.

Antioxidant levels diminish with age, therefore the ageing brain appears to be an easy target for oxidative damage. This underscores the importance of getting enough antioxidants through diet and supplements.

Antioxidant chemicals cooperate and network together. These cooperating chemicals include vitamin C, vitamin E, glutathione, coenzyme Q10, and lipoic acid. They actually revive and spare one another from destruction.

In his book, The Antioxidant Miracle, Dr. Packer gives an example of how this metabolic synergy works to protect cells. "When vitamin E disarms a free radical, it becomes a weak free radical itself. But unlike bad free radicals, the vitamin E radical can be recycled, or turned back into an antioxidant, by vitamin C or coenzyme Q10. These network antioxidants will donate electrons to vitamin E, bringing it back to its antioxidant state. The same scenario occurs when vitamin C or glutathione defuses a free radical," (Packer, 1999).

The main detoxification system that handles various toxins/poisons is called the Glutathione Conjugation Pathway. Glutathione heads the process by sticking to toxins and helping to transport them from your body in the form of faeces and bile.

A deficiency of glutathione may play a role in the development of many illnesses and diseases, including schizophrenia, cancer, infections and dementia. As you age, glutathione levels decrease, making it important to incorporate lifestyle choices that keep it steady.

<u>Stress, Nutrition and Immune Response</u>

Numerous research findings point to oxidative stress mechanisms as a common thread in various neurological and emotional conditions such as schizophrenia, depression, bipolar disorder, anxiety disorder, autism, dementia, multiple sclerosis and so on.

The link between nutrition and immunity also supports the role of antioxidants in mental health.

Recognition of immune system dysfunction in people with mental health conditions, particularly those with depression or schizophrenia, has led to different hypotheses for their pathogenesis, including infections and autoimmune factors.

Repairing the central nervous system is facilitated by both cellular and humoral components of the immune system and adequate nutrition (i.e. vitamins, minerals and antioxidants) supports these processes.

The impact of nutrition on the immune system is discussed further in chapter 8.

I WAS RESISTANT to medication as it gave me some horrendous side-effects; I didn't want to take it but I had nothing else, and no one was offering any alternatives. Instead I was told that I needed to be on the medication, that I couldn't be well without it, and that I'd need to be on medication for life.

The reason for such a drastic diagnosis was due, in part, to my family history of mental illness: both my mum and my brother have been on medication, are still on medication, and my mum has become institutionalised along with the medication. I didn't want to believe that would be my outcome and I was determined that things would be different for me. I just couldn't explain how.

Simply abandoning the medication caused terrible symptoms – worse than the illness itself – and resulted in my being readmitted on to a mental health unit and then sectioned when I resisted medication. With no professional support, combined with the fact that I was unable to convince even my family that medication was not the answer, I ended up feeling quite alone with my situation. I was determined, however, not to let it get the better of me.

Although there's constant talk of empowerment, there's such a major emphasis on medication it causes people to become disempowered. The treatment choices need to be opened up.

7   NEUROTRANSMITTERS, MEDICATION AND NUTRITION

One of the great benefits of nutrients and really paying attention to what you eat is the fact that your brain gets certain types of nutrients which may be needed to boost its neurotransmitter functions. For example, you may need something that works on dopamine and acetylcholine, because those are the two neurotransmitters that are responsible for the power and speed of your brain.

Nutritional deficiencies can cause problems in the absorption and assimilation of amino acids, proteins, essential fatty acids, vitamins and minerals that are needed to synthesise vital neurotransmitters. This can manifest as symptoms of inability to concentrate, poor ability to communicate, memory problems, depression and various other symptoms that show up when a person is not making proper neurotransmitters.

Examples   of   Neurotransmitters   and   Their
Functions

Neuro-transmitter & Function	Examples of malfunctions
Acetycholine (Ach) Enables muscle action, learning and memory	Alzheimer's Disease, Ach-producing neurons deteriorate
Dopamine Influences movement, learning, attention and emotion	Excess dopamine receptor activity linked to schizophrenia. Starved of dopamine, the brain produces the tremors and decreased mobility of Parkinson's disease
Serotonin Affects mood, hunger, sleep and arousal	Under-supply, linked to depression
Norepinephrine Helps control alertness and arousal	Under-supply can depress mood

GABA	Under-supply linked
(Gamma-aminobatyric acid)	to seizures, tremors and insomnia
A major inhibiting neurotransmitter	
Glutamate	Over-supply can over stimulate brain, producing migraines or seizures (which is why some people avoid MSG, monosodium glutamate, in food)
A major excitatory neurotransmitter involved in memory	

Neurotransmitter health must be maintained with a balanced diet that includes adequate amounts of protein, carbohydrates and fats. No food group can be eliminated, since they are all critical for proper neurotransmitter production and function. Dietary neurotoxins – like excess caffeine, nicotine and alcohol – decrease production and should be avoided (see Appendix A: *High Caffeine Use and Psychotic Symptoms – A Case Study*).

Nutrients and the Body

The human body requires 17 vitamins and 24 mineral elements; it contains about 54% to 70% water, 15% proteins, 14% to 25% fat, 5% to 6% mineral matter, and about 1% carbohydrates.

Carbohydrates (broad groups of food nutrients), although they represent the smallest proportion in the human body (about 1%), they make up the bulk of our diet and constitute the chief source of energy (about 70%).

Proteins are the major source of building material for the body and play an important role as structural constituents of cellular membranes. Proteins function in the maintenance and repair of worn tissues.

Enzymes, which are primarily proteins, are biological catalysts by the nature and amount of amino acids (essential amino acids), whilst **vitamins** can be considered as necessary nutrients, required for the proper utilisation of bulk nutrients-carbohydrates.

Furthermore, vitamins and **minerals** are the constituents of enzymes functioning as catalysts in the regulation of most biological processes.

A number of studies have shown that micronutrient deficiency may impair one or more critical brain functions, relating to mood-related psychiatric symptoms. When patients in research samples have multiple micronutrient deficiencies, single-nutrient interventions may show only marginal effects; multiple-nutrient interventions, however, result in more complete, dramatic effects. The concept of multiple-micronutrient deficiency may explain why clinical trials using single-nutrient interventions show only marginal effects.

Neurotransmitters

There are two main groups of neurotransmitters:

- **Excitatory** neurotransmitters/neuromodulators   (i.e.: uppers)

- **Inhibitory** neurotransmitters/neuromodulators   (i.e.: downers)

A proper balance between the excitatory and inhibitory neurotransmitters is essential; excitatory symptoms can be caused by either an excess of excitatory neuromodulators OR a deficiency of inhibitory neuromodulators.

Neurotransmitters operate in distinct systems made up of neurons communicating together in circuits, and require micronutrient cofactors in their synthesis.

Micronutrients play a key role in regulating neural transmission. For example, Folic acid and vitamin B_{12} are involved as cofactors in serotonin and norepinephrine synthesis; Thiamine serves as a coenzyme in acetylcholine; vitamin B_6 serves as a cofactor in the synthesis of the neurotransmitters dopamine, serotonin, norepinephrine, histamine, and GABA (vitamin B_6 deficiency has been shown to reduce brain production of serotonin and GABA).

Neurons and how they communicate

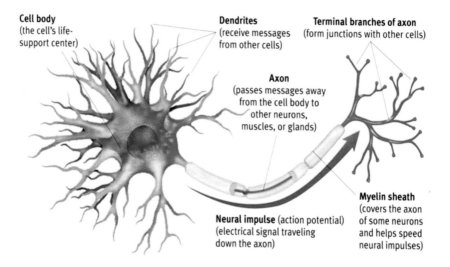

Cell body
(the cell's life-
support center)

Dendrites
(receive messages
from other cells)

Terminal branches of axon
(form junctions with other cells)

Axon
(passes messages away
from the cell body to
other neurons,
muscles, or glands)

Myelin sheath
(covers the axon
of some neurons
and helps speed
neural impulses)

Neural impulse (action potential)
(electrical signal traveling
down the axon)

Dendrites – 'listen' to things coming in from the outside i.e. touch or heat.

Axons – 'speak' by sending out (process and send out).

The cell sends the action potential when it reaches a threshold. The threshold is reached when excitatory ("Fire!") signals outweigh the inhibitory ("Don't fire!") signals by a certain amount.

Types of Neurons

Sensory neurons carry messages IN from the body's tissues and sensory receptors to the CNS for processing.

Motor neurons carry instructions OUT from the CNS out to the body's tissues

Interneurons (in the brain and spinal cord) process information between the sensory input and motor output.

The neuron receives signals from other neurons; some are telling it to fire and some are telling it to not fire. When the threshold is reached, the action potential starts moving. Like a gun, it either fires or it doesn't; more stimulation does nothing. This is known as the "all-or-none" response.

Next the action potential travels down the axon from the cell body to the terminal branches. The signal is transmitted to another cell. However, the message must find a way to cross a gap between cells. This gap is called the synapse.

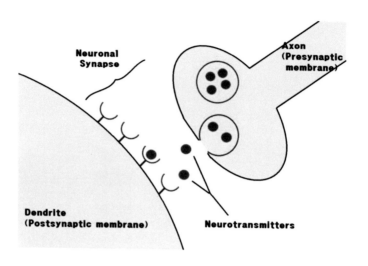

Impact of Anti-Psychotic Medications on Neurotransmitters

Most anti-psychotic drugs impact neurotransmitters by altering their activity. What this means is that anti-psychotics affect brain cell function by either exciting or inhibiting them, by the speeding up or slowing down of their activity.

All psychoactive substances, from socially acceptable drugs such as caffeine to anti-psychotic drugs such as clozapine, affect the activity of neurons, although each has its own potency, target in the brain, and psychoactive effect.

Anti-psychotic drugs in general interfere in the functioning of several neurotransmitters and receptors, notably dopamine. Many older anti-psychotic drugs show strong correlations between their ability to block dopamine receptors in the brain – particularly subtype D-2 – and their ability to relieve psychotic symptoms. For example, clozapine targets serotonin receptors more than it does dopamine receptors.

Dopamine receptors, like serotonin and other neurotransmitter receptors, are found in different parts of the brain and body. These receptors have different subtypes that are given numbers, such as D-1, D-2, D-3, D-4 and so on. Each subtype has a different function.

Dopamine D-2 receptors control body movements; if they are blocked the tremors associated with Parkinson's Disease can result. However, since anti-psychotics like clozapine has less of an effect on the D-2 receptors, it does not cause symptoms like Parkinson's Disease but it does have very strong anti-psychotic actions. It also interacts with other receptors, not only those specific to dopamine and serotonin. These interactions seem to account for some of the side-effects that may occur with clozapine, including drowsiness, constipation, difficulty urinating and possible weight gain.

Impact of Nutrients on Neurotransmitters

The body needs more than 20 amino acids in order to make all of the various chemicals used by the body. Eight of these amino acids are called essential because the body cannot make them on its own; they have to come from food. Examples of amino acid precursors for neurotransmitters include:

- 5-HTP $\rightarrow$ serotonin and melatonin
- L-Tryptophan $\rightarrow$ serotonin and melatonin
- L-DOPA $\rightarrow$ dopamine
- Choline $\rightarrow$ acetylcholine
- Glutamine $\rightarrow$ GABA
- GABA $\rightarrow$ inhibitory neurotransmitter that boosts overall brain chemical message function.

Certain micronutrients can affect the propagation of nerve impulses. In particular, adequate intake of both folate and vitamin B_{12} is important in maintaining the integrity of the myelin sheath (the insulating layer of tissue made up of lipids and proteins that surrounds nerve fibres, allowing rapid and efficient transmission of nerve impulses). Thiamin is needed for the maintenance of the nerve's membrane potential and for proper nerve conductance. Additionally, iron has an important role in the development of oligodendrocytes (the cells in the brain that produce myelin).

Vitamin C plays a role in synthesising dopamine and norepinephrine (it also protects your brain from oxidative damage).

B-complex-vitamin B_5 helps you make acetylcholine neurotransmitter, while vitamin B_6 aids in the production of serotonin. Both vitamins B_{12} and B_9 allow your brain to metabolise neurotransmitters, helping to control the levels of neurotransmitters found in your brain tissue.

Neurotransmitters, such as dopamine and serotonin, require a lot of building blocks in the form of amino acid precursors, that the body can take and put together to form more complex compounds.

A person cannot just take dopamine and serotonin as a tablet because they would be broken down by the stomach into their amino acid and other compounds, and never make it into the bloodstream intact.

The bottom line is that nutrients provide the naturally occurring building blocks for neurotransmitters.

A depletion in certain neurotransmitters can result in obesity, depression, anxiety, learning disorders and panic attacks.

NEUROTRANSMITTER MOLECULE:

THE KEYS THAT FIT PERFECTLY!

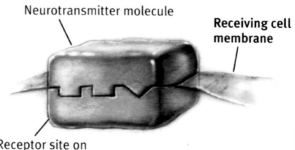

Neurotransmitter molecule

Receiving cell membrane

ESSENTIAL NUTRIENTS PRODUCES NATURALLY OCCURRING SUBSTANCES:

THE KEYS THAT FIT

Receptor site on receiving neuron

This neurotransmitter molecule has a molecular structure that precisely fits the receptor site on the receiving neuron, much as a key fits a lock.

A naturally occurring substance/neurotransmitter molecule has a structure that precisely fits to the receptor site on the receiving neuron, much like a key fits a lock.

How Anti-Psychotic Drugs Act On Neuron Receptors

One of the most fundamental concepts in pharmacology is based upon molecule-receptor interactions. Receptors are the specialised molecular binding sites where neurotransmitters dock, producing physiological effects.

This concept applies not only to the action of extrogenous substances like anti-psychotic drugs, but also to naturally occurring or endogenous substances such as neurotransmitters and hormones.

Many drugs mimic the effects of hormones and neurotransmitters because they bind with the same receptors as neurotransmitters. However, most anti-psychotics don't do anything completely new to the body. Rather they mimic or influence naturally occurring processes.

ANTI-PSYCHOTICS **THE KEYS THAT DON'T QUITE FIT!**

AGONIST **AND** ANTAGONIST **MOLECULES**

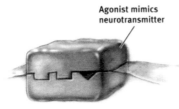

Agonist mimics
neurotransmitter

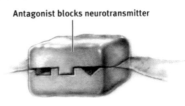

Antagonist blocks neurotransmitter

An agonist molecule fills the receptor site and activates it, acting like the neurotransmitter.

An antagonist molecule fills the lock so that the neurotransmitter cannot get in and activate the receptor site.

Anti-psychotics can only help to use up neurotransmitters that are already present, so without providing the essential nutrients depletion will take place.

This would explain why drugs that block reuptake of neurotransmitters can, in the long-term, further deplete neurotransmitters. An important point to note here is that drugs do not provide the body with the beneficial raw materials required to make more neurotransmitters, instead they cause neurotransmitters to remain longer in the synapse (between the dendrites), and these are then further broken down by enzymes. This can result in having to increase the dosage of the anti-psychotic drug or using a second drug because the first drug stops working after a time (most likely due to depleted neurotransmitters).

Understanding the 'Agonist' and 'Antagonist' Process of Anti-Psychotics

If a drug produces an effect to the same extent as the naturally occurring substance, it is called a full agonist. If a drug produces the same general response, but to a lesser effect than the naturally occurring substance it is a called a partial agonist. If a drug augments or facilitates an endogenous compound's effect without actually binding to the naturally occurring substance's receptor, it is referred to as an indirect agonist.

Anti-psychotic drugs can prevent endogenous compounds from binding to their receptors by occupying the receptor without producing a physiologic response. Such drugs are referred to as antagonists. As is the case with indirect agonists, if a drug diminishes or prevents an endogenous compound's effect without actually binding to the naturally occurring substances receptor, it is referred to as an indirect antagonist.

Furthermore, some drugs can also bind to a receptor and provoke an action opposite to that of the endogenous substance.   Such drugs are called inverse agonist.

Just like there are full and partial agonists, there are full and partial inverse agonists too, such as Pimavanserin (ACP-103) – a highly selective 5-HT2A inverse agonist (used for treating psychosis in Parkinson's Disease patients).

It's worth noting that drugs can inhibit enzymes from performing their physiologic activities or they can activate enzymes so that they become more active than usual. For example, a drug can inhibit an enzyme that is necessary to deactivate a neurotransmitter, thereby increasing or prolonging its activity (e.g. as a MAO-I drug used for depression).   Drugs can also block transporters or reuptake pumps that usually operate to recycle neurotransmitters.

Drugs can also cause more or less neurotransmitters to be released from axon terminals through various actions, such as causing more vesicles to release their contents upon depolarisation or by causing the vesicles themselves to become leaky, thus depleting their contents.

Also bear in mind that drugs can influence the degree that ion channels open or close in the cell membranes.

As you can see, drugs have multiple actions that produce not just the desirable therapeutic effect, but also side-effects as well.

Profiling the Adverse Effects of Anti-Psychotics

1st Generation Anti-Psychotics: *Higher risk of neurological side-effects*	The first generation anti-psychotics were associated with higher risks of neurological side-effects such as tardive dyskinesia, parkinsonism, muscle stiffness, autonomic dysfunction, dry mouth, and so on.
2nd Generation Anti-Psychotics: *Higher risk of metabolic side-effects*	The second generation anti-psychotics (SGAs) gained popularity due to a reduced risk of neurological side-effects, but later it was discovered that these drugs are associated with an increased risk of developing metabolic side-effects, such as diabetes mellitus, hypoglycaemia, weight gain, atherogenic lipid profile and so on.

Second generation anti-psychotic drugs (SGAs) are a group of medications used to treat some psychiatric conditions, such as schizophrenia, acute mania, bipolar disorder and other mental conditions. SGAs are also referred to as 'atypical' anti-psychotics. The term 'atypical' refers to the fact that they generally do not cause the same degree of movement side-effects that are common to the first generation, or so-called 'typical' anti-psychotics.

Examples of first generation anti-psychotics include:

- Chlorpromazine
- Haloperidol
- Perphenazine, and
- Trifluoperazine

Examples of SGAs include:

- Clozapine
- Olanzapine
- Risperidone
- Paliperidone, and
- Quetiapine

The use of SGAs is common nowadays as a treatment for psychosis, however there are increasing concerns about their related metabolic side-effects.

The adverse risk factors are not only for cardiovascular disease, insulin resistance and diabetes mellitus (leading to increased morbidity and mortality), but also that they impair the patients' adherence to treatment. SGAs, in particular are associated with significant weight gain, with clozapine and olanzapine carrying the highest risk.

Most prescription drugs, including commonly used antidepressants, lead to side-effects. This usually discourages patients from taking medication. Such non-compliance is a common occurrence encountered by psychiatrists.

Consequently, a consensus development conference convened issuing recommendations on patient monitoring when treated with SGAs.

According to a number of patients, psychosocial consequences of weight gain, such as a sense of demoralisation, physical discomfort and being the target of substantial social stigma are so intolerable that they may discontinue treatment, even if they think the treatment is effective. The clinical importance of preventing excessive weight gain is paramount, as excessive weight gain poses serious health risks. This makes treatment of anti-psychotic drug induced metabolic disturbances as important as the actual treatment of psychotic illnesses.

"...the increased prevalence of these chronic conditions is due to multiple factors, but it has become clear that certain anti-psychotics – particularly some of the newer anti-psychotics, mood stabilizers, and antidepressants – contribute to the increased risk of obesity."
(Ganguli, 2012)

Medications and Nutrient Deficiencies

The knowledge that long-term use of medication leads to nutritional deficiencies of specific nutrients has been well documented by a large number of studies done over the last three decades. Conclusively, these studies have shown that medications deplete nutrients – whether by interfering with absorption, or by inhibiting transport or metabolism. Yet this information is not generally communicated to the people taking the medications. In a nutshell: Nutrients are essential to the metabolic activities of every cell in the body (Becker, 2010).

According to a recent study: Folate and Vitamin B_{12} can reduce the disabling symptoms in some patients:

"The symptoms of schizophrenia are complex, and anti-psychotic medications provide no relief for some of the most disabling parts of the illness. These include negative symptoms, which can be particularly devastating," says Joshua Roffman, MD. MMSc. of the MGH Department of psychiatry. "Our finding that folate plus vitamin B_{12} supplementation can improve negative symptoms opens a new potential avenue for treatment of schizophrenia. Because treatment effects differed based on which genetic variants were present in each participant, the results also support a personalised medical approach to treating schizophrenia."

"Folate (or folic acid) is required for the synthesis of DNA and neurotransmitters, as well as in gene expression."
(Roffman, et al., 2013).

Combining therapies to maximise success: Getting serious about choice, recovery and personalisation.

"Giving patients more choice and more control in their healthcare is an essential part of the Government's work to put the NHS on the side of the patients. No two people are the same, which is why our plans offer patients more personalised care, ensuring that 'no decision about me is made without me'."
(Howe, 2012).

There is good evidence that 'personalised' nutritional therapy plays an important role in addressing both mental and physical health problems, including metabolic syndromes.

What is Metabolic Syndrome?

Metabolic syndrome is a collection of risk factors that are associated with increased morbidity and mortality due to type 2 diabetes mellitus and cardiovascular disease. One of the most important underlying risk factors is abdominal obesity and insulin resistance.

Second generation anti-psychotics cause more significant changes in the metabolic parameters, increasing the chances of developing metabolic syndrome and associated disorders like diabetes mellitus, obesity, cardiovascular disorders, insulin resistance and so on. For example, the olanzapine anti-psychotic drug has the maximum potential to cause metabolic syndrome.

Patients may have multiple components of the metabolic syndrome, whether or not they are overweight or obese.

Nutrition has effects on whole-body metabolism and its regulation, via effects on hormones, transcription factors and lipid metabolic pathways. Nutritional components of the diet regulate the metabolic health of an individual either by controlling the expression of some key genes related to metabolic pathways or by modulating the epigenetic events on such genes.

Nutrition deficiencies are often a contributor to metabolic syndromes; when these deficiencies are identified and fixed, amazing results have been shown.

Detoxifying the body from built up toxins has also proved beneficial. For example, uncleared toxins from medications can end up being stored in brain and nerve tissues. Hence, the toxins left behind need to be removed in order to create the conditions for optimal states of health to occur.

Nutrition Therapy Works Side By Side with Medications

"...we know that choice over the type of treatment you receive and involvement in joint care planning are also critical to a person's recovery."
(Farmer, 2012).

Combined use of prescription medications like SSRIs with nutrient therapy has shown therapeutic advantages. Up to date studies suggest that adding dietary precursors boosts the production of neurotransmitters, while the medications allow more efficient use of them. This combined treatment approach may permit lowering of medication dosages.

Bear in mind that most of the excess mortality in persons suffering from schizophrenia is attributed to physical illness, with cardiovascular illness being a major contributor.

A cornerstone of management strategy in such patients is the use of nutrients to nourish the cells, decrease body weight, and improve glycaemic control and cardiovascular risks.

The Government's Mandate to the NHS Board makes clear the commitment to giving mental health equal importance with physical health, in all relevant aspects of the NHS.

"By giving patients more choice in their care, we are making sure they get the right type of high quality mental health care... which suits them and their needs... a further step to make sure they have more choice, more control and more information about their care."
(Lamb, 2012).

The Department of Health has put forward measures to give patients more involvement, greater control and choice over their care.

Commissioners and care providers can reflect/echo genuine commitment to meeting the Department of Health's strategic guide for improving outcomes by:

- Providing patients with greater choices/options for engaging in nutritional educational programs and therapies. This will offer patients (including carers, families and friends) greater opportunities for meaningful involvement at all stages. Patients will have greater control/self-management, and be empowered with a greater sense of independence whilst taking on a more active role/involvement in their care and treatment.

- Acknowledging and valuing nutritional therapy (along with other current therapies such as Cognitive Behavioural Therapy) as the overarching piece in a very complex jigsaw puzzle related to holistic health/recovery.

SOME PEOPLE ARE quite happy to take medication, maybe because, for them, the side-effects are not so severe. For others, the side-effects are so horrendous that they'd rather suffer and try something else. That was me; I was desperate.

I was prepared to try anything, and I now realise that that is the sort of desperation that many people feel about being forced with medication and, as a result, forced to remain in the system. This 'treatment' is actually counterproductive.

Whenever a person is resistant to something – upset or angry etc. – the body produces certain types of chemicals in preparation for stress: the fight/flight response. After a prolonged period, these chemicals can produce negative effects on the body. So, the angrier I became at having to be forcibly treated with medication etc., the more unwell I was becoming. The "treatment" wasn't making me well, in fact, with a combination of the side-effects along with my resistance, medication was exacerbating the very condition it was supposed to be curing!

Long-term medication combined with stress is destructive, as the research on telomeres has shown; biological ageing increases rapidly, as does the risk of co-morbidity. Both the ageing process and psychological stress are interactive; each can dysregulate immune function, altering the responsiveness of the nervous and immune system.

Can Stress Really Wreak Havoc on both the Mind and Body?

Interplay between the immune, nervous and endocrine systems is most commonly associated with the pronounced effects of stress on immunity.

Is there a way in which your thoughts – how you think about your life, how you think about yourself – are able to influence the immune system? How does the brain 'talk' to the immune system and how does the communication take place? And what about stress? Is it true that stress can influence your immune system?

It's one thing to say that the mind can affect the immune system but it's another thing to say a disease could actually be affected as a result.

Why do we care about the immune system? Why do we care that the brain affects hormones that influence and alter the distribution and function of immune cells in the body?

I think we care because the immune system plays a vital role in a variety of diseases.

We know that when we are under stress we experience certain emotions that are registered in the brain. That's an easy, well understood relationship between the brain and the immune system. We also know that brain scans show a different pattern of activity in the brain when you're angry than when you're afraid.

So the brain is our channel for affecting the body in response to different emotional signals and different thoughts. And the brain triggers the release of hormones into the body, including stress hormones.

There is a particular pathway in the body that starts in the brain, in a particular region of the brain called the hypothalamus that triggers the release of a cascade of hormones, or factors, that end up with the release of stress hormones such as cortisol. The hypothalamic neurons can trigger the release of a variety of intermediating substances including norepinephrine and epinephrine.

Hypothalamic neurons can also trigger activation of the ANS (autonomic nervous system).

Stress hormones circulating in the body – because your brain is experiencing, for example, a fear or stress reaction – can influence what gets dumped into the bloodstream (glucose and fatty acids) and what happens to various organ systems (increased heart rate and digestive system shut-down) when your sympathetic nervous system gets aroused.

These hormones (cortisol, norepinephrine and epinephrine) can then affect the immune system; the distribution of immune cells and their functions. Meaning they affect where your immune cells go (where they migrate to in the body).

Stress hormones circulating in the body can not only influence where your immune cells go, they can also influence the functioning of those cells. So they can alter the way the immune cells are able to act; the way immune cells can kill bacteria, for example. Stress hormones are very powerful in that they can influence movement of these cells and they can influence their activity.

Where Are Immune Cells?

White blood cells (leucocytes) are cells that can be found everywhere in the body; in the bloodstream, blood vessels, lymphatic vessels and so on. The lymphatic vessels shadow along the blood vessels and are the channel for leucocytes – the way in which the leucocytes travel throughout the body.

At certain points along those lymphatic vessels reside lymph nodes packed with leucocytes. There's a lot of activity against viruses and so on happening right there inside the lymph nodes, and these are found in the neck, under the arms and in a variety of other places in the body.

There are far more immune cells in the gut than in any other place in the body, protecting us from organisms that we may ingest. The gut is in fact a large immune organ, and the gastrointestinal tract is referred to as the largest immune system in the body. There are also immune cells present in bone marrow.

One of the things that stress hormones can do is they can act on leucocytes and cause them to move differently throughout the body. This movement is called 'trafficking', and leucocytes traffic differently when there's an outpouring of stress hormones. For example, they go to the lymph nodes, which then act like battle stations when you're under stress, as if the immune system is preparing for the body to be wounded.

Stress and the Immune System

Part of what our bodies are wired to do is traffic those cells to places that they're going to be most useful in an emergency. One of the really important ways that stress affects the immune system is just by moving those cells into different locations, which enables them to be more effective.

But it's not just moving the cells here and there in the body. As mentioned before, the stress hormones also change activity of the cells.

T-cells are leucocytes that are able, for example, to kill cells that are infected with a virus. Each T-cell is programmed to respond only to a very narrow range of foreign organism. The first thing they do when they come into contact with something foreign is to divide and proliferate. This is so that they can create an army of the same type of T-cells, all capable of fighting that particular organism. Stress hormones can suppress this proliferation response and down-regulate it (dampen it down).

Stress hormones can also act on B-cells, another type of leucocyte. B-cells produce antibody molecules (proteins) that attach to and neutralise invaders such as bacteria, for example.   Stress hormones reduce the antibody production ability of these B-cells.

Another type of leucocyte, known as the 'natural killer cell', is capable of killing tumours; potentially playing a very important role in the body. They can also kill viral infected cells, but they don't require specificity; natural killer cells will kill any type of virus. These used to be called promiscuous cells because they were so non-selective they would go after any foreign organism. Stress hormones can also suppress the functioning of these natural killer cells.

How they do this is by influencing the production of signalling molecules. The immune system is made up of all these different kinds of cells, and the way they work together is that there are these signalling molecules (cytokines, previously lymphokines) that orchestrate their activity. The fact that stress hormones can influence the production of key cytokines has quite wide ranging effects along various pathways.

One of the pathways is that the brain can trigger the release of stress hormones into the bloodstream, for example. Those hormones can then act on leucocytes of various types and cause them to redistribute or alter their function. So, by the stress hormones acting on the leucocytes these stress hormones can in fact be immune suppressive.

Another pathway is a neural pathway – meaning nerve fibres directly from the brain acting on leucocytes. This is a very quick system; you don't have to wait for a molecule to get somewhere slowly. This pathway is activated when an immediate threat is perceived; the heart starts to race and the sympathetic nervous system gets activated (almost instantly). That release from the sympathetic fibres can influence the activity of leucocytes via these neural pathways.

<u>Built For Stress</u>

Each one of those immune organs – the gut, the lymph nodes, the thymus and spleen – is innervative, meaning there are neural fibres entering into them. What are these neural fibres – that enter the immune organs directly from the brain – doing?

When scientists look at these organs, they find these fibres right next to leucocytes (they're super close to leucocytes), and when the sympathetic nervous system gets activated it releases the hormone norepinephrine right into those immune organs, next to those leucocytes. Norepinephrine acts on the leucocytes inside the immune organ – for example, the lymph node – by acting on receptors on the leucocyte for norepinephrine. Clue number one that the body was built to respond to stress! Leucocytes have receptors built specifically to respond to a norepinephrine signal; a stress hormone signal.

Clue number two is that the brain is able to communicate directly with the immune system; the brain influences what the leucocytes in the lymph nodes do. This is very important because most of the fight between immune cells and, for example, viruses is not taking place in our bloodstream, it's taking place in the lymph nodes and the immune organs, and that's getting modified and altered by the release of stress hormones.

Studies have indicated that immune dysfunction may be an underlying pathophysiological mechanism contributing to mood disorders, including schizophrenia and major depression.

The Inflammatory Response and Mental Health

Cytokines, which regulate immune function, may influence the central nervous system and play a key role in mediating depression-like neurobehavioural changes.

It has been established that physiological concentrations of pro-inflammatory cytokines that occur after infection, act in the brain to induce common symptoms of sickness, such as loss of appetite, sleepiness, withdrawal from normal social activities, fever, aching joints and fatigue. This syndrome has been defined as sickness behaviour.

The fact that cytokines act in the brain to induce physiological adaptation, leads to the hypothesis that inappropriate, prolonged activation of such cytokines through immune dysfunction may be involved in a number of pathological disturbances in the brain. Specifically, pro-inflammatory cytokines have been associated with alterations in neurotransmitter balance, and hence a number of psychological disorders.

Interferon alpha (interferons are particular cytokines) has been associated with confusion, apathy, anxiety and depression. Long-term, increased levels of interferon alpha may lead to down-regulation of dopamine and depletion of serotonin.

Interferon gamma may specifically promote the degradation of tryptophan, leading to reduced synthesis of serotonin and hence play a role in depression (Wirleitner, Neurauter, Schröcksnadel, Frick, & Fuchs, 2003).

Stress and Inflammation: Culprits of Disease?

Psychological stress is associated with greater risk for depression, heart disease and infectious diseases, but until now it has not been exactly clear how stress influences disease and health.

Sheldon Cohen (Professor of Psychology at the Carnegie Mellon University, Pennsylvania) argues that prolonged stress alters the effectiveness of cortisol to regulate the inflammatory response, because it decreases tissue sensitivity to the hormone. Specifically, that immune cells become insensitive to cortisol's regulatory effect. In turn, runaway inflammation is thought to promote the development and progression of many diseases.

"Inflammation is partly regulated by the hormone cortisol and when cortisol is not allowed to serve this function, inflammation can get out of control."
(Dr. Cohen, 2012)

In his research, published in National Academy of Sciences, Professor Cohen showed for the first time how the effects of psychological stress on the body's ability to regulate inflammation can promote the development and progression of disease.

"The immune system's ability to regulate inflammation predicts who will develop a cold, but more importantly it provides an explanation of how stress can promote disease. When under stress, cells of the immune system are unable to respond to hormonal control, and consequently, produce levels of inflammation that promote disease. Because inflammation plays a role in many diseases such as cardiovascular, asthma and autoimmune disorders, this model suggests why stress impacts them as well. Knowing this is important for identifying which diseases may be influenced by stress and for preventing disease in chronically stressed people," (Dr. Cohen, 2012).

Chronic Stress and Oxidative Damage

Sustained negative stress is now acknowledged as a key driver behind many of today's health complaints, both psychological and physical.

Because the term "stress" has long been used incorrectly, it has lost its medical meaning; people often use the term to describe any situation they don't like. For this reason, neuroscientists have recently clarified the term to mean:"...conditions where an environmental demand exceeds the natural regulatory capacity of an organism, in particular situations that include unpredictability and uncontrollability," (Koolhaas, et al., 2011).

Chronic negative stress triggers a number of critical changes throughout the body that act along multiple biochemical pathways, including the endocrine, nervous, and immune systems.

When stress is severe, chronic, or multi-layered, numerous biochemical changes overwhelm the body's homeostatic mechanism i.e. "...environmental demand exceeds the natural regulatory capacity." Studies have found that these harmful effects can persist long after a stressful situation has been normalised (Opstad, 1994); (Esterling, Kiecolt-Glaser, Bodnar, & Glaser, 1994).

As a result, key biochemical levels can remain for too long at suboptimal levels (Epel, 2009). This is called 'homeostatic imbalance'.

Some of the many disease states associated with stress-induced homeostatic imbalance include:

- Obesity
- Diabetes
- Osteoporosis
- Hypertension
- Cardiovascular Disease
- Infectious disease
- Gastric ulcer
- Cancer
- Gastrointestinal complaints
- Skin issues
- Neurological disorders
- Sexual dysfunction
- Psychological problems
- Suppressed immunity
- Reduced telomerase and shortened telomeres
- Accelerated cellular and tissue ageing (as a result)

(Wikgren, et al., 2012); (Epel, 2009); (Houben, et al., 2009); (Watfa, et al., 2011); (Tchirkov & Lansdorp, 2003)

Whatever the stressor, the cascade of physiological responses is the same.

First, within seconds of the stressful event, various chemicals—neurotransmitters and hormones such as cortisol – are released into the bloodstream. They launch the initial fight-or-flight, stress-adaptation responses in which blood glucose rises, blood vessels constrict, the heart races, and blood is diverted away from the digestive system. These responses originate at the cellular level and within every key body system, including the neuroendocrine system, the hypothalamus-pituitary-adrenal (HPA) axis, the immune system, and the primary (endogenous) antioxidant enzyme system.

Second, within minutes of the stressful event – and possibly lasting for several hours, weeks, or longer – specific biochemical pathways are activated within these systems, disrupting the body's natural homeostasis. If the body cannot restore equilibrium quickly, permanent damage occurs. The end result is a vast spectrum of chronic diseases.

The biochemical effects of stress can be complicated and diverse, but basically, they contribute to the development of or create imbalance in the following:

- Cortisol (steroid hormone)
- Neurotransmitters (noradrenalin, dopamine, serotonin, acetylcholine, GABA)
- Hypothalamus-pituitary-adrenal (HPA) axis regulation
- Glucose (blood sugar)
- Primary antioxidant activity (e.g., superoxide dismutase, catalase)
- Immune activity

- Amyloid (linked to 20 serious diseases including Alzheimer's)
- Inflammation (e.g., cyclooxygenase, or COX enzyme)
- Gastric ulcerations
- Lipid peroxidation (e.g., hepatic)
- Plasma creatine kinase (enzyme)
- ATP (adenosine triphosphate)
- Cognition and memory function
- Sexual response and function

(Downey, 2012)

Innate Immune System Pathological Role in Psychiatric Disorders: What's the Evidence?

There is by now substantial clinical evidence for an association between specific mood disorders and altered immune function. More recently, a number of hypotheses have been forwarded to explain how components of the innate immune system can regulate brain function at the cellular and systems levels and how these may underlie the pathology of disorders such as depression, PTSD (Post-Traumatic Stress Disorder) and bipolar disorder.

Pathophysiological studies in schizophrenia were focused on disturbances of the dopaminergic neurotransmission over decades without convincing results; antipsychotic anti-dopaminergic drugs still show unsatisfactory therapeutic effects. New concepts in the biological research of schizophrenia are therefore required.

Recently, genetic data from multiple large groups of patients were published in 'Nature' showing that different gene loci located on chromosome 6p22.1 are the most probable susceptibility genes for schizophrenia (Shi, et al., 2009); (Stefansson, et al., 2009); (Purcell, et al., 2009).

The region includes several genes of interest, which are related to the immune function. The strongest evidence for association was observed in or near a cluster of histone protein genes which could be relevant through their roles in regulation of DNA transcription or repair, i.e. in epigenetics (Costa, et al., 2007), or their direct role in antimicrobial defence (Kawasaki & Iwamuro, 2008). Moreover, several genes of the HLA (Human Leucocyte Antigen) complex, which regulate the immune function and are involved in schizophrenia, are located in these regions (Fellerhoff, Laumbacher, Mueller, Gu, & Wank, 2007).

There is no doubt that the dopaminergic neurotransmission plays an important role in the pathophysiology of schizophrenia. Although the role of dopamine in schizophrenia has been intensely studied, the exact underlying pathological mechanisms are still unclear.

Dopaminergic hyperfunction in the limbic system and dopaminergic hypofunction in the frontal cortex are discussed to be the main neurotransmitter disturbances.

Recent research provides further insight that glutamatergic hypofunction might be the cause for this dopaminergic dysfunction in schizophrenia (Swerdlow, van Bergeijk, Bergsma, Weber, & Talledo, 2009).

The function of the glutamatergic system is closely related to the immune system and to the tryptophan-kynurenine metabolism, which both seem to play a key role in the pathophysiology of schizophrenia (Müller & Schwarz, 2007); (Müller & Schwarz, 2007b).

Tryptophan-kynurenine metabolism is basically metabolism of tryptophan via the kynurenine pathway – a metabolic pathway involved in physiological functions such as behaviour, sleep, thermoregulation and pregnancy.

Infection during pregnancy in mothers of offspring who later develop schizophrenia has been repeatedly described, in particular in the second trimester (Brown, et al., 2004); (Buka, Goldstein, Seidman, & Tsuang, 2000). As opposed to any single pathogen, the immune response, itself, of the mother may be related to the increased risk for schizophrenia in the offspring (Zuckerman & Weiner, 2005). Indeed, increased IL-8 levels of mothers during the second trimester were associated with an increased risk for schizophrenia in the offspring (Brown, et al., 2004).

A five-fold increased risk for developing psychoses later on, however, was detected after infection of the CNS in early childhood (Brown, et al., 2004); (Gattaz, Abrahão, & Foccacia, 2004). These data were confirmed in recent studies (Koponen, et al., 2004); (Brown A. S., 2008); (Dalman, et al., 2008).

Importance of Understanding the Biological Basis: The Body Lives and Functions as a Whole!

"The fact that every organ in the body exists and works in contact with the rest gets forgotten. The body lives and functions as a whole, where every system, organ, tissue and even cell depend on each other, affect each other and communicate with each other. One should not look at, let alone treat, any organ without taking the rest of the body into account."
(Campbell-McBride, 2004)

Understanding the biological basis for mental illness is extremely important to combat the stigma attached mental illness.

- There are a range of mental illnesses and many seem extremely dissimilar. Mental illness may seem distinct from physical illness because it is easy to think of the mind as separate from the body. However, the brain functions like any other bodily organ; the brain needs certain hormones, chemicals and nutrients at certain levels, and, just like with any other organ, imbalances can lead to symptoms and disorders.

MY JOURNEY THROUGH mental illness has been quite complex, because at the very beginning I didn't know what the journey would be like. I didn't acknowledge that I was experiencing a mental illness because it took so many forms that at times it did take me by surprise. Where I thought I knew what the manifestation of symptoms would be, they would come in a different form, which I believe led to the different diagnoses.

At the core of it, whatever the diagnosis is – of which I've had a few – is how you address it. Although I'd been given these different diagnoses, I dealt with them through nutrition. That tells me that whether you're suffering from psychosis and hearing voices, or you're delusional, manic, or seriously depressed; nutrition can address all of those things.

During one of the last episodes I had – episodes which at times I hid from my family and from my doctor for fear of ending up back on a mental health unit – I was staying with my daughter and her family and I was becoming extremely paranoid. However I wanted to put into practice what I'd learned about nutrition over time. It was real hard work, but I was determined, so I made a number of requests for various things.

As I say, it was one of the last episodes I had.

Most people are aware and have a basic understanding of the connections between nutrition and physical health. On the other hand only a few people seem to be aware of or understand the connection between nutrition and mental illness. However, nutrition can play a key role in the onset, severity and duration of many mental disorders.

The most common mental disorders that are currently prevalent globally are depression, bipolar disorder, schizophrenia and obsessive compulsive disorder. The dietary intake pattern of these populations is often deficient in many nutrients, especially essential vitamins, minerals and omega-3 fatty acids.

A notable feature of the diets of those suffering from mental disorders is the severity of deficiency in these nutrients. Essential nutrients are often effective in reducing patients' symptoms because nutrients are converted to neurotransmitters which in turn alleviate depression and other mental health problems.

The most common nutritional deficiencies seen in patients with mental disorders are of omega-3 fatty acids, b-vitamins, minerals and amino-acids. Amino-acids act as precursors to neurotransmitters.

Link between Psychological/Psychiatric Conditions and Omega 3: What's the Evidence?

(See also Appendix B: *Evidence for Link between Psychological/Psychiatric Conditions and Omega-3*)

Children
• Learning and behaviour • Dyslexia • Dyspraxia • ADHD symptoms
Five 'negative' studies* No benefits for unselected ADHD population found in: • Two studies using DHA (Voigt, et al., 2001); (Hirayama, Hamazaki, & Terasawa, 2004), • One using pure EPA (Gustafsson, et al., 2010) • Two using a combination (Johnson et al., 2008; Matsudaira et al., 2008). **Abstract** (Gustafsson, et al., 2010) CONCLUSIONS: Two ADHD subgroups (oppositional and less hyperactive/impulsive children) improved after 15-week EPA treatment. Increasing EPA and decreasing

Omega-6 fatty acid concentrations in phospholipids were related to clinical improvement.

*NB: Two of these RCTs report benefits for particular subgroups.

Five 'Positive' Studies

Significant benefits for children with:

- Dyslexia
- Dyspraxia and/or
- ADHD type symptoms

Found in:

- Studies using both EPA and DHA (Richardson & Puri, 2002); (Stevens, et al., 2003); (Richardson & Montgomery, 2005); (Sinn & Bryan, 2007); (Vaisman, et al., 2008).

RCT of dietary supplementation with fatty acids in children with developmental coordination disorder (Richardson & Montgomery, 2005).

117 underachieving children aged 5-12 years from mainstream schools:

- All showed specific difficulties in motor coordination (DSM-IV DCD)
- 40% were behind expected achievement in reading and spelling

- Over 30% scored in the clinical range for ADHD-type symptoms (> 2SD above population means)

Abstract

CONCLUSIONS: Fatty acid supplementation may offer a safe efficacious treatment option for educational and behavioural problems among children with DCD. Additional work is needed to investigate whether our inability to detect any improvement in motor skills reflects the measures used and to assess the durability of treatment effects on behaviour and academic progress.

Adults

- Self-harm
- Borderline Personality Disorder
- Anxiety Disorders
- Stress/hostility and aggression
- Age-related cognitive decline
- Alzheimer's Disease (early stage)

In each case, pilot RCTs have provided some preliminary evidence of possible benefits.

Summary (Mahadik, Pillai, Joshi, & Foster, 2006)

Evidence is increasing for increased oxidative stress and cell damage in schizophrenia. Furthermore, treatments with some anti-psychotics together with the lifestyle and dietary patterns, that are pro-oxidant, can exacerbate the oxidative cell damage and trigger progression of neuropathology. Therefore, adjunctive use of dietary antioxidants and EPUFAs, which are known to regulate the growth factors and neuroplasticity, can effectively improve the clinical outcome. The dietary supplementation of either antioxidants or EPUFAs, particularly omega-3 has already been found to improve some psychopathologies. However, a combination of antioxidants and omega-3 EPUFAs, particularly in the early stages of illness, when brain has high degree of neuroplasticity, potentially may be even more effective for long-term improved clinical outcome of schizophrenia.

The Neglected Link Between Eating Disturbances and Aggressive Behavior in Girls
(Thompson, Wonderlich, Crosby, & Mitchell, 1999)

Abstract

CONCLUSIONS: Eating disturbances are significantly associated with aggressive conduct in adolescent girls. The constellation of eating disturbances and aggressive behaviour is associated with a greater risk of drug use and attempted suicide.

Recommendations from international scientific and health organisations

- General population – cardiovascular health: ≥ 500mg/day EPA + DHA (Cunnane, Drevon, Spector, Sinclair, & Harris, 2004); (Brenna, Salem, Sinclair, & Cunnane, 2009).
- Depression or other health conditions: ≥ 1000mg (1g)/day EPA + DHA (Freeman, et al., 2006); (Hibbeln & Davis, 2009).

Highlighting the Importance of Essential Fatty Acids

In the UK, US, Australia and Canada, most people consume less than 150mg/day.

EPA and DHA are both essential and they have different but complementary roles.

All natural foods that contain these key omega-3 fatty acids provide both of them together.

Humans show limited conversion of EPA to DHA, and little or no conversion of DHA to EPA.

Ideal ratios may vary with age and condition:

- Possibly more DHA than EPA for young infants or pregnant mothers
- Possibly more EPA than DHA for mood disorders

Fish and seafood provide other essential nutrients that few other foods contain.   In addition to providing long-chain omega-3 (EPA and DHA), fish is also an important dietary source of other nutrients important for brain function including:

- Vitamin D
- Iodine
- Selenium

Key nutritional issues in disorder of mood, behaviour and cognition:

- Blood sugar regulation problems
- Fatty acid deficiencies/imbalances
- Micro-nutrient deficiencies/imbalances
- 'Anti-nutrient' and toxicity issues
- Food allergies/intolerances
- Gut dysbiosis/digestion and malabsorption issues

Artificial Food Colouring and Hyperactivity (Food Standards Agency UK)

But it's not only about what we're not eating, disorders can also be triggered by what we <u>are</u> eating. Research funded by the FSA has suggested that consumption of mixes of certain artificial food colours and the preservative sodium benzoate could be linked to increased hyperactivity in some children.

The artificial colours are:

- sunset yellow FCF (E110)
- quinoline yellow (E104)
- carmoisine (E122)
- allura red (E129)
- tartrazine (E102)
- ponceau 4R (E124)

A European Union-wide mandatory warning must be put on any food and drink (except drinks with more than 1.2% alcohol) that contains any of the six colours. The label must carry the warning 'may have an adverse effect on activity and attention in children'.

<u>What Are the Key Messages being Conveyed from these Research Findings and Evidences?</u>

- Nutrition matters to brains as well as bodies
- Nutrition is not an alternative approach – it is fundamental
- Controlled trials show benefits for mood, behaviour and cognition from some dietary interventions such as:
  - Supplementation with long-chain omega-3 fatty acids
  - Withdrawal of artificial food colourings
- Modern Western-type diets are NOT healthy and are affecting the way our brains develop and function
- The issues are not just about obesity and poor physical health

- Nutrition affects mental health and performance throughout life, so it's worth getting the basics right.

Nutrition and Anti-Social Behaviour

For a more convincing analysis of cause and effect, an Oxford University team led by nutritionist and criminologist Bernard Gesch has been investigating how the diet of young men in prison affects their propensity to violence.

Funded by the Wellcome Trust, the ambitious three-year research study is tracing the effect that nutritional supplements have on levels of violence for over 1,000 inmates, between the ages of 16-21 held at Polmont, Scotland, and two other British prisons.

The Randomised Controlled Trial of dietary treatment of 231 young offenders imprisoned at a high security unit in the UK entailed giving each prisoner either a multi-vitamin and fatty acid supplement, or a matched placebo.

Gesch's is the first large scale research project to attempt to unpick this relationship using experimental methods. It will also be a "double-blind" trial, meaning that neither the participating prisoners nor the prison staff knew whether they were handling nutritional supplements or a harmless placebo.

Influence of Supplementary Vitamins, Minerals and Essential Fatty Acids on the Antisocial Behaviour of Young Adult Prisoners. Randomised, Placebo-Controlled Trial. (Gesch, Hammond, Hampson, Eves, & Crowder, 2002)

Abstract

CONCLUSIONS: Antisocial behaviour in prisons, including violence, are reduced by vitamins, minerals and essential fatty acids with similar implications for those eating poor diets in the community.

The study goes further, using regular blood sampling to assess physiological processes that occur because of nutritional deficiency.

"The idea of a link between diet and anti-social behaviour is not a new one," says Gesch.

Gesch's study is designed to settle the question of whether there is a link between poor diet and violence, at least among prison populations. The policy implications, though far reaching, would be fairly straightforward: feed prisoners a balanced diet, low in sugar and processed foods, with nutritional supplements.

But why stop at prisoners? Whilst the setting - where what inmates eat is tightly controlled and where participants are more likely to demonstrate obviously violent behaviour - provides fertile ground for an experimental study, the results may hold water beyond the prison walls.

ONE OF MY first experiences of mental illness happened back in the 1980's, but I didn't end up in the mental health system at that time. It began with a sensation of having or carrying a heavy weight on my head, and I found myself walking and stooping as though I was trying to stoop under the weight of something.

At that time I realised something was wrong but I didn't know what it was. I went to the doctor and was given tranquilisers. The tranquilisers didn't address any of the issues and eventually I attempted suicide. Of course, I didn't really want to take my life; it was a cry for help, but at the same time I felt that I would have gone ahead and done it even though I didn't want to.

The tranquilisers gave me an altered sense of self; I could carry on as if everything was fine but I was actually going through a lot of emotional problems. I didn't realise that I was experiencing depression because I didn't feel depressed. I would wonder why I kept shedding tears but could not stop myself from crying and would feel embarrassed about it. Other times I just felt as though I could sleep and never wake up because this was a way to escape the reality and a way of easing the stress.

Nutrition helped me to rebuild, balance and strengthen the neurological connections between my brain and body.

A sustained poor diet can lead to depression and is a leading cause of disability worldwide.

Depression is a serious illness and is characterised by sustained sadness and loss of interest along with psychological, behavioural and physical symptoms.

Unlike the occasional sadness everyone feels due to life's ups and downs, depression profoundly weakens your ability to function in everyday situations by affecting your:

- Mood
- Thoughts
- Behaviour, and
- Physical well-being

The exact cause of depression remains unclear but it's thought that elements including a persons' genetics, the balance of chemicals in the brain and the environment a person lives in, may be involved. There also appears to be a psychological element to depression. However, it's most likely that depression isn't caused by any one thing. Instead it may well be the end result of a combination of influences.

Taking a Closer Look at the Elements:

Genetics

Depression appears to run in families, which suggests that genetics play a part in a person developing the condition.

Brain chemical imbalance

You may have also heard that depression is caused by an imbalance of certain chemicals in the brain called neurotransmitters. These neurotransmitters allow brain cells to communicate with each other by sending and receiving messages. These are the same chemicals that many of the current depression medications affect. Because of this, it can be assumed the neurotransmitters have an impact on depression.

What is not clear is whether a chemical imbalance plays a part in causing depression or if the imbalance occurs as the result of a person being depressed.

Environment

Environmental factors also appear to play a role in a person developing depression.

The loss of a loved one, chronic illness, stress at work or home, or unwelcomed life changes, can often trigger a depressive episode – even in individuals without a family history.

Psychological factors

Furthermore, psychological factors may influence a person's likelihood for developing depression. This includes things such as poor coping skills, negative thinking and judgement problems.

Common Symptoms of Depression

Sad, gloomy, dejected, downcast – these are some of the terms used to define depression in the dictionary. We all experience these feelings from time to time, but does it mean that we are or have clinical depression?

Not necessarily!

A number of specific symptoms must be present before a diagnosis of clinical depression is made. And this will depend on how long the symptoms have been present.

If a person has five or more of the following 11 symptoms for two weeks or longer, a diagnosis of depression may be made. These symptoms include:

- A persistent sad, anxious, or empty mood
- Feelings of hopelessness and pessimism
- Feelings of guilt, worthlessness and helplessness
- Loss of interest or pleasure in activities such as a hobby or interest that used to be enjoyed, including sex

- Decreased energy, fatigue and being slowed down
- Difficulty concentrating, remembering or making decisions
- Insomnia or over-sleeping
- Change in appetite or eating patterns such as eating much less or much more or a significant weight loss or gain.
- Restlessness and irritability
- Thoughts of death, suicide or suicide attempts
- Persistent physical symptoms that do not respond to treatment, such as headaches, digestive disorders and chronic pain.

Keep in mind that having some signs of depression does not necessarily mean that you are clinically depressed. For example, it is not unusual to feel restless or irritable when living with the stress of particular issues such workload, loss of employment, financial or family problems.

Up to a point such feelings are simply a part of human experience. It's only when these symptoms continue for an unusual length of time or increase in intensity, that there is good reason to suspect that what appeared to be a temporary mood has turned into depression.

It's important to understand that clinical depression is not something that you can WILL AWAY. You can't just pull yourself together and get better.

Clinical depression is serious and if it's left unaddressed, it can last for weeks, months or sometimes even years.

Evidence of the Links between Food and Depression

A growing body of evidence links eating patterns with an increased risk of depression.

Research shows that there are many variables associated with diet and mood, and that dietary patterns, specific foods and nutrients can impact your brain and mood.

The following studies highlight the impact of food on depression:

Researchers reported in the British Journal of Psychiatry in 2009 that a processed foods diet – rich in processed meat, sweet desserts, fried food, refined cereals and high-fat dairy – is a risk factor for depression in middle-aged people, compared with a whole foods pattern that is rich in vegetables, fruit and fish.

Another study in 2010, also published in the British Journal of Psychiatry, found that a dietary pattern characterised by vegetables, fruit, lean meat, fish and whole grains was associated with lower odds for major depression than the typical Western diet of processed or fried foods, refined grains and sugary products.

Most of us are becoming aware that diets high in processed foods and low in plant foods promote chronic, low-grade inflammation. These diets are implicated as a contributing factor in heart disease, diabetes and even some cancers. Now researchers are exploring how this diet also impacts depression.

Scientists from the University of Pittsburgh Medical Centre reported in the November 2011 Journal of Rheumatology that compelling evidence suggests that inflammation contributes to the development of depression. Many depressed people have higher levels of inflammation in their bodies, which appears to promote depression through many biological pathways.

It has now been recommended that adherence to a traditional Mediterranean style diet, which includes fruits, vegetables, nuts, cereals, legumes, fish and olive oil will also help protect against depression.

This diet provides abundant phytochemicals, omega-3 fatty acids, fibre, B vitamins and antioxidants – all of which are considered to be anti-inflammatory.

But the studies go even further:

Can eating fish protect against suicide and depression?

Japanese researchers found that a diet high in fish protects people from depression and suicide. A Finland team of researchers surveyed 1,767 residents and concluded that eating fish more than twice a week has a protective effect against suicide and depression (see also Appendix E: *Suicide Attempts Linked to Inflammatory Chemical*).

Other significant research has identified that people who are depressed may have low levels of positive neurotransmitters – brain chemicals – like serotonin and dopamine. These are sometimes referred to as the "feel good" brain chemicals.

Lots of medications used to treat depression specifically target raising serotonin (such as SSRIs).

Serotonin is the neurotransmitter most directly linked to depression although other neurotransmitters, like dopamine, can make people feel good.

Serotonin is the relaxing and calming neurotransmitter, whereas dopamine is the energetic neurotransmitter.

The brain uses the amino acid tryptophan to make serotonin. Tryptophan is widely distributed in protein-rich foods such as meat, poultry and fish, but the other amino acids in those foods interfere with the entry of tryptophan into the brain which results in the brain's inability to make adequate serotonin.

This is where eating a "balanced" diet comes in. So for example, eating carbohydrate foods such as whole grains, fruits, legumes and starchy vegetables along with protein foods enables tryptophan to get into the brain.

When you eat carbohydrates, your body digests and absorbs them and blood glucose levels rise. In response, insulin levels rise, which ushers glucose from your blood into your body's tissues, and also moves some of the competing amino acids from the blood into muscle tissue.

This mechanism helps open a passage for tryptophan to enter the brain and be converted to serotonin.

As with so many other diseases it's not just about focusing on specific nutrients, it's about focusing on a well-balanced diet of nourishing, whole foods; foods that raise blood sugar in a controlled way and help tryptophan get across the blood brain barrier.

Link between Fast Food and Depression Confirmed

According to a recent study headed by scientists from the University of Las Palmas de Gran Canaria and the University of Granada, eating commercial baked goods (fairy cakes, croissants, doughnuts, etc.) and fast food (hamburgers, hotdogs and pizza) is linked to depression.

Published in the *Public Health Nutrition* journal, the results reveal that consumers of fast food, compared to those who eat little or none, are 51% more likely to develop depression.

Furthermore, a dose-response relationship was observed. In other words "the more fast food you consume, the greater the risk of depression," explains Almudena Sánchez-Villegas, lead author of the study.

With regard to the consumption of commercial baked goods, the results are equally conclusive. "Even eating small quantities is linked to a significantly higher chance of developing depression," as the university researcher from the Canary Islands points out.

Increasing Alertness

Eat protein-rich foods to boost alertness, such as foods rich in protein i.e. turkey, tuna and chicken – which are rich in an amino acid called tyrosine. Tyrosine helps boost levels of the brain chemicals dopamine and norepinephrine. This boost helps you feel alert and makes it easier to concentrate.

Nutrients that May Help Ease Depression

Vitamins/Minerals/Enzymes

*Vitamin B-group, *Vitamin B12 (i.m.), *Zinc, *Calcium, *Magnesium, *Lecithin, *Lithium (may have side effects)

Amino Acids/Fatty Acids

*Amino acid group, *L-Tyrosine, *GABA, *Taurine, *Flax-oil, *Hemp oil, *Primrose oil, *Blackcurrant oil

Food/Herbs and other recommendations

*St. John's Wort, *Kava Kava, *Liquorice root, *Burdock root, *Ginkgo biloba, *Regular walks, good company, watching and reading comedies to shift your attention

Avoid

*Sugar, *Alcohol, *Saturated fats, *Heavy meals, *Junk food

Foods to eat

*Carrots, *Beetroots, *Asparagus, *Broccoli, *Spinach, *Pumpkin, *Sweet potatoes, *Seeds, *Nuts, *Fish (eg. Salmon, mackerel and tuna), *Turkey, *Apricots, *Bananas, *Blueberries, *Kiwis, *Oranges

Foods to avoid

*Processed/refined foods, *Sugars, *Caffeine, *Fast foods, *Fried foods, *Alcohol, *Drugs

Considerations and precautions

*Clinical studies show the amino acid tyrosine and the b-vitamins aid all forms of depression,

*Caution: if taking MAO inhibitor drugs, avoid L-tyrosine, *Food allergies and certain drugs have been linked to depression. Omitting certain foods really helps, *Insufficient complex carbohydrates may cause serotonin depletion and depression. Hypoglycaemia and thyroid disorders are often causes. Heredity is also a factor, *Hormonal imbalances may be behind depression, *Melatonin, a helpful brain hormone, is released by bright light and sunlight – avoid dark rooms.

Association between Depression and Omega-3: What's the Evidence?

Across countries, rates of depression are inversely related to seafood consumption.

Within countries, individuals consuming less fish and seafood are more likely to become depressed.

Patients with depression have lower blood concentrations of omega-3 found in fish and seafood.

Randomised Controlled Tests of Omega-3 for Mood Disorders
In adults: Five recent 'meta-analyses' show significant benefits for depression (including bipolar disorder). American Psychiatric Association recommends > 1g/day

EPA + DHA as an add-on treatment for mood disorders (Freeman, et al., 2006). Mixed results from studies including more varied population and treatments (Appleton, et al., 2006); (Rogers, et al., 2008).

In children:

One pilot RCT to date, showing significant benefits for children with depression (Nemets, Nemets, Apter, Bracha, & Belmaker, 2006).

American Psychiatric Association treatment recommendations:

- All adults should eat fish at least 2 times per week.
- Patients with mood, impulse control or psychotic disorders should consume 1g/day of EPA + DHA
- A supplement may be useful in patients with mood disorders (1-9g/day). Use of > 3g/day should be monitored by a physician.

NB: These recommendations are in addition to standard treatments for psychiatric disorders (not as a substitute) (Freeman, et al., 2006).

"UK dietary surveys show that average fish intakes are well below the recommended two portions per week. Given that the majority of consumers do not eat oily fish, it is reasonable to consider the potential

contribution of dietary supplements or fortified foods…"
(Ruxton & Derbyshire, 2009).

MY SECOND EXPERIENCE came some years later after giving birth; emotional trauma, such as the trauma of childbirth is one of the triggers for mental illness. I remember feeling very different from how I felt normally, and that I was having a lot of thoughts that weren't quite rational.

I started to feel very high and elated, and at the time it felt good, as if I was on some kind of drug – even though I never partook in drugs. I realise that this is what is referred to as mania.

One of the reasons, I believe, that people who experience mania will embrace the feeling is because it's a feel-good feeling. You feel as though life is fantastic and as if you can do all kinds of things. You may even feel that you have special abilities.

I was so full of energy that I began to think that everyone else was dead and only I was alive. This delusion became worse over time as I found that the mania stopped me from sleeping.

I also experienced another extreme. Where I felt so depressed that I believed I was dead and that everyone else was alive, and when anyone was talking to me it seemed to be from a distance because I believed that I wasn't real any more but that I was in fact some kind of spirit.

What Is Bipolar?

Bipolar is a brain disorder that involves periods of depression followed by elevated moods or mania (in the absence of drugs or alcohol). Normal moods may be experienced between these mood shifts, which can be mild or severe and the changes may occur gradually or quickly. This illness is also known as manic depression and is a serious illness.

The mood swings that accompany bipolar disorder are unlike the typical ups and downs that people sometimes experience as a normal part of life. They are intense and can negatively impact the person being affected. These fluctuations in mood can be dramatic enough to lead to risky behaviour, damaged relationships and/or careers, the inability to function and may even lead to suicidal tendencies if left unaddressed.

It is said that bipolar disorder is a medical illness caused by a chemical imbalance in the brain. This illness is real; it is not just a thought or feeling that can be dismissed by the person affected. It is not a sign of weakness or failure. Although the exact cause of bipolar disorder is unknown, research suggests that a genetic predisposition is involved.

Both men and women appear to be affected equally by bipolar disorder. Approximately one per cent of the general population is at risk for cyclic bouts of depression and mania. Young people are at the highest risk for bipolar disorder, as the first episode often occurs between the ages of 15 to 25. Sometimes, however, the first episode may not occur until many years later.

Symptoms of Mania or Manic Episodes

- Increased or excessive energy, activity, and restlessness, increased interest in activities
- Excessively high, overly good, euphoric mood
- Extreme irritability
- Racing thoughts and talking very fast, jumping from one idea to another
- Rapid, unpredictable emotional changes
- Distractibility, inability to concentrate well
- Reduced or no sleep needed
- Unrealistic beliefs in one's abilities and powers, inflated self-esteem
- Poor judgment
- Spending sprees
- A lasting period of behaviour that is different from usual
- Increased sexual drive, sexual indiscretions
- Abuse of drugs, particularly cocaine, alcohol, and sleeping medications
- Provocative, intrusive, or aggressive behaviour

- Denial that anything is wrong
- Overreaction to stimuli, misinterpretation of events

Mania can include different states, such as hypomania, severe mania or hyper-mania, and psychosis.

Hypomania

Hypomania is a mild to moderate level of mania, which may feel good to the person experiencing it as they may become highly functional and productive. People experiencing hypomania are often very pleasant to be around due to their positive mood, intense interest in other people and activities. Unable to recognise this positive mood as something to be concerned about, it is not uncommon for the person affected to deny anything is wrong. This can be dangerous however, as hypomania can develop into severe mania or can just as easily switch into a severe depression.

Severe Mania or Hypermania

Hypermania exceeds the usual spectrum of a manic episode and can lead to paranoia, hyper-sexuality (resulting in sexual promiscuity and sexual risks), reckless behaviour, and overspending.

Psychosis

Psychosis, such as hallucinations (hearing, seeing, or sensing things that are not actually there) and delusions (false beliefs not influenced by logical reasoning or cultural concepts), may sometimes occur. Usually during psychosis, the person experiences a euphoric mood and the unrealistic sense of great self-importance or grandiosity.

Symptoms of Depression (with Bipolar Disorder)

- Sad mood
- Preoccupation with failures or inadequacies and a loss of self-esteem
- Feelings of uselessness, hopelessness, excessive guilt
- Slowed thinking, forgetfulness, difficulty in concentrating and in making decisions
- Loss of interest in work, hobbies, people
- Social isolation
- Lethargy
- Agitation/irritability
- Changes in appetite or weight (eating too little or too much)
- Changes in sleep (sleeping too little or too much)
- Decreased sexual drive
- Suicidal thoughts

A depressive episode is diagnosed if five or more of the above symptoms last most of the day, nearly every day, for a period of 2 weeks or longer.

The depressive cycle experienced by someone with bipolar disorder is very similar to major depressive illness, however, people with bipolar disorder often feel more irritable than depressed. There is also a tendency towards too much sleep when in the depressed cycle, rather than insomnia, which is more typical of major depression. Weight gain is also more common to people with bipolar disorder as opposed to weight loss, which is fairly common among depressed people.

According to the Diagnostic and Statistical Manual of mental disorders: The criteria for diagnosing bipolar disorder contains 3 components:

1. Major depressive episode
2. Manic and hypomanic episode
3. Mixed episodes

The ICD-10 Classification of Mental and Behavioural Disorders by the WHO, provides diagnostic guidelines for:

- Manic episode
- Hypomania
- Mania with or without psychotic symptoms
- Depressive episode
- Mild and moderate depressive episodes and
- Severe depressive episodes with and without psychotic symptoms

Bipolar disorder is found in all ages, races, ethnic groups and social classes, with an equal number of men and women being affected. According to the National Institute of Mental Health, if one parent has bipolar disorder, the likelihood of you developing this illness is

15 to 30 per cent. This risk increased to between 50 and 75 per cent when both parents have the illness. However, only a fraction of those individuals who are at genetic risk actually do acquire the illness. Also of interest is that 20 per cent of adolescents with major depression develop bipolar disorder within a five-year period of experiencing their first depressive episode.

Evidence Implicating Inflammatory Mediators in the Pathophysiology of Bipolar Disorder and Major Depression.

Signs of a link between bipolar illness and inflammation can be seen in biochemical analysis of brain specimens obtained at autopsy. Researcher Rapaka Rao in the laboratory of Stanley Rapoport at the National Institute on Ageing at the National Institutes of Health in Bethesda, Maryland, has reported that increased markers of neuronal inflammation and excitotoxicity were found in the brains of people who had had bipolar disorder.

"Bipolar disorder is associated with neuroprogression, and oxidative stress, neurotrophins, and inflammation may underpin this process."
(Dr. Berk, 2011).

"Early interventions can potentially improve the outcome" of bipolar disorder, "and the new findings give new opportunities to find effective neuroprotective agents."
(Dr. Berk, 2011).

Bipolar Affective Disorder is associated with increased production of pro-inflammatory cytokines both in the manic and in the depressed phase as compared to healthy subjects. This is the first study, which examined both mania and bipolar depression (O'Brien, Scully, Scott, & Dinan, 2006).

Increased Oxidative Stress in Bipolar Disorder

When energy is created within cells, toxic by-products can accumulate and potentially damage cells. This process is known as oxidative stress, and the toxins created include peroxides, nitrates, and free radicals.

Keila Ceresér and colleagues reported increases in serum levels of thiobarbituric acid reactive substances (TBARS) in patients with bipolar disorder. TBARS are indicators of damage to cells' lipid membranes, and carbonyl is a measure of protein oxidative damage. These findings were replicated by Brisa Fernandes and colleagues, who found increases in TBARS during mania.

"We increasingly think there is a systemic biology that underpins bipolar disorder and potentially other inflammatory diseases. The brain does not exist in isolation, and we need to understand that pathways similar to those that underpin risks for cardiovascular disorders, stroke, and osteoporosis might also underpin the risk for psychiatric disorders, and that other treatments might be helpful."
(Dr. Berk, 2011).

Both inflammation and oxidative stress increase risk of cardiovascular disorders, and patients with mood disorders are said to lose 10 or more years of life expectancy from cardiovascular disorders compared to the general population. Research also suggests that inflammation and oxidative stress may contribute to the symptoms, evolution, and progression of the mood disorders themselves.

Nutrition and Bipolar Disorder Research Findings

Folic acid

Folate deficiency is the most common nutrient deficiency and may be found in over ¼ of hospitalised psychiatric patients (Lipton, Mailman, & Numeroff, 1979); (Källström & Nylöf, 1969); (Hunter, Jones, Jones, & Matthews, 1967).

Folate deficiency is associated with a wide variety of psychiatric symptoms including depression as well as neurological symptoms of weakness, numbness, stiffness and spasticity, both with and without muscular atrophy (Howard, 1975).

A team from Israel measured homocysteine levels in 41 bipolar patients and found, "Patients who show functional deterioration have plasma levels of homocysteine which are significantly elevated as compared with controls." They add that bipolar patients without deterioration had homocysteine levels which were almost identical to the non-bipolar group.

Homocysteine can be effectively lowered by increasing intake of folic acid.

Vitamin B$_{12}$

Observational study: Patients admitted to a Norwegian mental hospital were measured for serum B$_{12}$ levels during a 1 year period. It was estimated that the percentage of hospitalised mental patients with below normal levels of vitamin B$_{12}$ was 30 times higher than in the general population (Edwin, Holten, Norum, Schrumpf, & Skaug, 1965).

Vitamin C

Observational study: The average plasma vitamin C level in 885 psychiatric patients was 0.51/100 ml compared to 0.87/100 ml in 110 healthy controls. 32% of the patients had levels below 0.35 mg/100 ml, the threshold which has been associated with detrimental effects on immune responses and behaviour (Schorah, Morgan, & Hullin, 1983).

Observational study: Anxiety and excitement were found to increase the rate of breakdown of ascorbic acid (Maas, Gleser, & Gottschalk, 1961).

Observational study: Over 10% of 465 hospitalised psychiatric patients in Essex, England showed delayed ascorbic acid saturation (seventh day of loading or later) which indicates borderline or actual scurvy. Most of these patients had obvious clinical signs of the scorbutic state (Leitner & Church, 1956).

Experimental Double-blind Crossover Study: 23 hospitalised bipolar patients (11 manic, 12 depressed) were rated as to symptoms, given ascorbic acid 3 gm or placebo, and rated hourly for the next 6 hours. The next day, the procedure was repeated except that ascorbic acid and placebo were switched. The severity of illness fell slowly during the day in the placebo group, but much more rapidly in the treated group, with significant differences at 3, 4 and 5 hours post-ingestion (Naylor & Smith, 1981).

Calcium

Observational Study: Plasma calcium was lower in 11 manic patients than in 10 healthy controls (Bowden, et al., 1988).

Case Report: A 35 year old woman with no history of mania, but previously diagnosed as having a 'depressive character disorder' was admitted for treatment of an organic mental disorder associated with hypocalcemia and hypomagnesemia secondary to short bowel syndrome. Her bowel disorder required ongoing electrolyte replacement therapy, with which she was sometimes non-compliant.

Confusion and distractibility resolved rapidly with calcium and magnesium replacement. However, the patient soon became sleepless and euphoric, with pressured speech, increased psychomotor activity, racing thoughts, and feelings of immense power, but with a clear senorium. The manic syndrome lasted for 6 days and resolved without psychoactive drugs (Groat & Mackenzie, 1980).

Decrease in cerebrospinal fluid (CSF) calcium accompanies mood elevation and motor activation in depressed patients undergoing treatment with ECT, lithium, and total sleep deprivation. Similarly, decreases in CSF calcium occur during acute psychotic agitation or mania, while periodic recurrences of such agitated states are initially accompanied by transient increases in serum calcium and phosphorus. Such serum ion shifts trigger more enduring and opposite shifts in CSF calcium and, in turn, the manic behaviour (Carman & Wyatt, 1979).

Note: The overwhelming majority of calcium within cells resides in intracellular stores; free intracellular calcium accounts for <0.1% of total cell calcium content but has more direct consequences for cell excitability and may be more sensitive to subtle perturbations (Dubovsky, et al., 1989).

Potassium Chloride

Supplementation may eliminate some of the adverse side-effects of lithium treatment.

Experimental Study: 4 consecutive patients with lithium-induced polyuria (receiving 900-1200 mg lithium daily) were treated with potassium chloride twice daily. The mean 24 hr. urine volume dropped from 3.85 to 2.62 litres, while mean urine osmolality increased from 239 to 361 mOsm/L. Patients reported appreciable improvements in subjective symptoms, including thirst and lithium tremor. Serum potassium rose by 0.14 mEq/L, while the serum lithium level was unchanged (Tripuraneni, 1990).

L-Tryptophan

6-12 gm in divided doses ((2wk. Trial) above 4 gm if combined with niacinamide).

Possible indications:

1. **For treatment of mania.**
   Experimental double-blind study: 24 newly admitted manic patients were treated for 1 week with 12 gm daily; then ½ the patients (chosen at random) continued on tryptophan while the other ½ received placebo. In the open phase, there was a clinically and statistically significant reduction in manic symptom scores. During the second week, only patients switched to placebo tended to show an increase in manic symptom scores (Chouinard, Young, & Annable, 1985).

   Experimental Double-blind Crossover Study: 5 patients typically received in random order L-tryptophan 6 gm with pyridoxine 50 mg for 2-3 weeks and chlorpromazine 400 mg with pyridoxine 50mg for 2 weeks. Ratings on the Sainsbury scale, while not significantly different, favoured L-tryptophan over the first 13 days, and chlorpromazine on most items over days 23-32. At the end point (day 34) L-tryptophan was favoured on all Sainsbury subscales except hostility. Results suggest that L-tryptophan may be equivalent to 400 mg chlorpromazine for the treatment of mania (Prange, Wilson, Lynn, Alltop, & Stikeleather, 1974).

Experimental Double-blind Study: 10 actively manic or hypomanic patients were given an average dose of 9.6 g tryptophan/d; 7 improved. 3 of the 7 relapsed when placebo was substituted for tryptophan under double-blind conditions (Murphy, et al., 1974).

2. **Potentiates effects of lithium in bipolar patients.**
Experimental Double-blind Study: Compared to 5 bipolar patients who received lithium alone, the combination of lithium and L-tryptophan (3 gm, 3 times daily) resulted in significantly greater improvement in 4 bipolar patients (Brewerton & Reus, 1983).

3. **Treatment for patients with bipolar II illness.**
Case Report: A 63 year old female failed to respond to imipramine and lithium but responded well to a trial of L-tryptophan alone for 11 months (Beitman & Dunner, 1982).

Food Sensitivities

Case Report: Marion, a 32 year old art teacher, had a 10 year history of severe mood swings diagnosed as manic depression. Lithium controlled her severe mood swings, however she felt very depressed and lethargic. Nutritional evaluation revealed mild magnesium and zinc deficiencies, but supplementation with these nutrients made little difference in her mental state.

She was then started on a diet restricted to fruit, vegetables, rice, meat and fish. After a month she felt distinctly less depressed and had few mood swings. After 2 months she had increased her work from 2 days a week to 4, and her friends and colleagues had noticed a remarkable improvement in her mood and in her previously glum appearance. Three days after eating bread, however, she became severely depressed and had to stop work for 6 weeks. She returned to her strict diet, and her depression cleared in 6-8 weeks (Davies & Stewart, 1987).

Observational Study: Anti-bodies to a variety of foods, especially cereals, were measured in serum from 100 patients with acute psychosis and 100 elective surgical patients as controls. There was an association between a possible secondary mania and the presence of IgE anti-bodies to wheat or rye (Rix, Ditchfield, Freed, Goldberg, & Hillier, 1985).

Blood Sugar

The more uneven your blood sugar supply the more uneven your mood.

Eating lots of sugar is going to give you sudden peaks and troughs in the amount of glucose in your blood; symptoms that this can cause include fatigue, irritability, dizziness, insomnia, excessive sweating (especially at night), poor concentration and forgetfulness, excessive thirst, depression and crying spells, digestive disturbances and blurred vision. Since the brain depends on an even supply of glucose it is no surprise to find that sugar has been implicated in aggressive behaviour, anxiety, depression, and fatigue.

Lots of refined sugar and refined carbohydrates (meaning white bread, pasta, rice and most processed foods) are also linked with depression because these foods not only supply very little in the way of nutrients but they also use up the mood enhancing B vitamins – turning each teaspoon of sugar into energy needs b-vitamins. Sugar also uses up other important nutrients.

The best way to keep your blood sugar level even is to eat what is called a low Glycemic Load (GL) diet and avoid, as much as you can, refined sugar and refined foods, eating instead whole foods, fruits, vegetables, and regular meals. There are a number of books that explain the low-GL diet in detail including the Holford Low GL Diet Bible. Caffeine also has a direct effect on your blood sugar and your mood and is best kept to a minimum. Also alcohol and drugs make all of the symptoms of bipolar disorder worse, creating a vicious cycle, ultimately triggering either full blown mania or depression.

Magnesium

Magnesium is interesting in bipolar disorder because of its chemical similarity to lithium (lithium being the drug most commonly used as a mood stabiliser). In fact, there is some evidence that the drug lithium may attach to the places inside the cell where magnesium is supposed to attach. In studies, some people with bipolar disorder or other psychiatric illnesses had differences in the amounts of magnesium in their blood (Chouinard, Beauclair, Geiser, & Etienne, 1990); (Giannini, Nakoneczie, Melemis, Ventresco, & Condon, 2000). There have been some studies where magnesium was added to other treatments to stop symptoms of mania or rapid cycling. Magnesium can block the entry of too much calcium into cells (it is a natural calcium channel blocker) which may explain why it is helpful with some symptoms of illnesses. Magnesium's role in supporting good sleep may also be quite important here, since many people with bipolar disorder experience increasingly poor sleep patterns preceding a manic episode.

Omega-3 Fatty Acids

Six double-blind placebo controlled trials of omega-3's and depression, five of which show significant improvement. The first trial by Dr Andrew Stoll from Harvard Medical School, published in the

Archives of General Psychiatry, gave 40 depressed patients either omega-3 supplements versus placebo and found a highly significant improvement. The next, published in the American Journal of Psychiatry, tested the effects of giving twenty people suffering from severe depression, who were already on antidepressants but still depressed, a highly concentrated form of omega-3 fat, called ethyl-EPA versus a placebo. By the third week the depressed patients were showing major improvement in their mood, while those on placebo were not. The latest trial by Dr Sophia Frangou from the Institute of Psychiatry in London gave a concentrated form of EPA, versus placebo, to 26 depressed people with bipolar disorder and again found a significant improvement. This may be because omega-3s help to build your brain's neuronal connections as well as the receptor sites for neurotransmitters; therefore, the more omega-3s in your blood, the more serotonin you are likely to make and the more responsive you become to its effects.

FINDING A CURE for my mental illness was always my focus, because obviously I wanted to be well. It was not just about managing the symptoms. So, with that in mind I was looking to find out what I could do to help myself without having to be on medication for life.

I had to look at whatever was easiest for me; obviously I can't make pharmaceutical medications myself, so food was the thing I looked at, since food is there to nourish the body.

We all eat food and we all need nutrients – there's no medication that can nourish the cell. All medications need food, in fact, as it's the nutrients in food that support the system that medication needs to work. The priority is for people to give their bodies the right nutrients – not necessarily to dismiss medication – but it should not be the be all and end all.

So I started to look at what kinds of foods I could eat, what kinds of supplements I could take; I wanted to learn about all of it, so I started to learn about nutrition.

We can all experience anxiety at some point in our lives; worrying about certain things is only natural. The problem occurs when we constantly worry, perhaps over a period of months, about a particular problem, never giving our body and mind a rest.

This in turn can then bring on feelings of anxiety for no real reason, creating more problems than the very thing we were first worrying about.

An anxiety disorder may lead to social isolation. It may also impair a person's ability to work and carry out routine activities.

It can also cause people to have trouble sleeping and create feelings of constant fatigue. In addition, there are many emotional problems to cope with: depression, constant worry and feelings of unreality.

It is at this point that most people reach for help. Examples of common anxiety disorders include:

Panic Disorder

People who suffer with panic disorders can suffer severe attacks of panic which may make them feel like they are having a heart attack or are going crazy – for no apparent reason. The desire to run away from the situation they are in is immense. Symptoms include a racing heart, sweating, trembling, feelings of dread, a fear of dying, fear of losing control, and feelings of unreality.

Generalised Anxiety Disorder (GAD)

GAD can occur with excessive, unrealistic worry over a long period of time. The anxiety may focus on issues such as health, marriage, money, career or any of the other worries the life of this world can present us with. In addition to chronic worry, GAD symptoms include trembling, muscular aches, insomnia, depression, feelings of unreality and irritability.

Social Anxiety Disorder

Social anxiety disorder is a form of anxiety created from a fear of what other people may think. Sufferers find it hard to cope in social situations; they become easily embarrassed, going beyond just shyness. They have little confidence and can be highly sensitive to what others think about them. This form of anxiety may lead to avoidance behaviour. The physical symptoms related to this form of anxiety can include a racing heart, faintness, blushing and excessive sweating.

Anxiety is a common problem that can be triggered by a number of factors and some research suggests that the tendency to become anxious may be inherited, and that some people learn to be anxious as a result of their upbringing.

Nevertheless, anxiety may be triggered by a combination of factors. For example, by an event that occurred in the past or a current problem, or by use of illicit drugs. Poor diet and caffeine may also trigger anxiety.

Common symptoms of general anxiety include:

- Disturbed sleep and tiredness
- Difficulty concentrating
- Expecting the worst in every situation
- Feelings of paranoia
- Feeling irritable
- Dizziness or faintness
- Nausea and stomach upsets
- Sweating
- Chest pains
- Rapid or heavy breathing
- Irregular heartbeats

Panic Attacks

Panic attacks occur when some of the physical symptoms of anxiety build up rapidly, and they may be accompanied by fears that you will have a heart attack, pass out or lose control.

Cycle of anxiety and fear leading to Panic Attack:

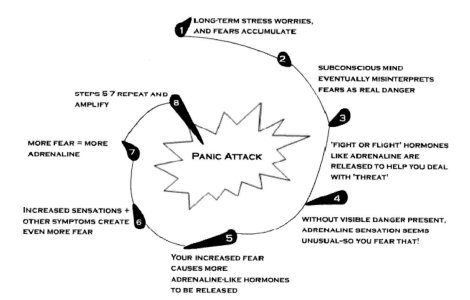

Nutrients that may help ease anxiety:

Vitamins/Minerals/Enzymes

*Vitamin B-group, *Calcium, *Magnesium, *Potassium, *Chromium, *Vitamin C, *Inositol

Amino Acids/Fatty Acids

*GABA, *DL-Phenylalanine, *L-Glutamine, *L-Tyrosine, *L-Glycine

Food/Herbs and other recommendations

*Herbs (hops, kava-kava root, St. John's wort, valerian root), *Regular walks, *Relaxation therapy, *Hot bath followed by a cold shower

Avoid

*Alcohol, *Nicotine, *Sugar, *Food and colour additives, *Drugs, *Bad company

Foods to eat	Foods to avoid
Yogurt	Fizzy drinks
Bananas	Processed food
Vegetables	White bread
Wholegrain foods	Chips
Brown Rice	Pastry
Beans	Cakes
Turkey	Caffeine
Chicken	Sugar
Cottage Cheese	Alcohol
Fresh Fish	Chocolate
Poached Egg	Cheese
Tuna	Fast Food
Fruit	
Porridge	
Baked potato	
Peanut butter	
Garlic	
Spinach	

Sources of nutrients that may help ease anxiety:

B vitamins: leafy green vegetables, whole grains, eggs, poultry, milk, soybeans

Vitamin C: oranges, papaya, strawberries, cantaloupe melon, kiwi fruit, bell peppers, parsley, broccoli, Brussels sprouts, kale

Magnesium: pumpkin, sunflower seeds, sesame seeds, leafy green vegetables

Complex carbohydrates: oatmeal, whole-grain breads, brown rice, sweet potatoes, carrots, green vegetables

Healthier fats: omega-3 fatty acids can be found in oily fish (salmon, mackerel, herring and light tuna), walnuts, flaxseed, beans, tofu, and olive oil; monounsaturated fats are another good choice and can be found in avocados, almonds, cashews, and peanuts

Lean protein: fish, shellfish, skinless chicken or turkey, loin or tenderloin cuts of red meat, low-fat or fat-free dairy, egg whites, egg substitutes, beans, legumes, tofu, soymilk

Tryptophan: poultry, milk, bananas, oats, cheese, nuts, peanut butter, sesame seeds.

DUE TO THE fact that I had experienced a range of psychoses – paranoia, hearing voices, etc., - my diagnosis was changed numerous times to: schizophrenia, paranoid schizophrenia, and schizoaffective disorder, to name a few, and strong emotions have been a trigger for my episodes.

I found that anger could trigger or increase my symptoms of psychosis. Whenever I got very angry, an overwhelming feeling of disorientation would engulf me. I would feel myself losing control as the anger and disorientation built up to such a degree that my brain and chest felt about to burst open. Unable to eat or sleep, the confusion, fear, paranoia and delusions would start (perhaps I'm being set up or something!). During my stays in hospital, and after being forced with medication, my symptoms would often get worse as my anger about the situation increased.

When emotional changes such as anger, elation or sadness occur, certain hormones are released within the body. This is natural, but some people already live with an imbalance of these hormones. Nutrition is a way that a person can affect some of the adjustment that is needed to bring balance about in the first place, and again after illness.

13 SCHIZOPHRENIA

Schizophrenia is a chronic, severe, and progressively disabling disorder of the brain. People with schizophrenia often suffer terrifying symptoms such as hearing voices not heard by others, or believing that other people are reading their minds, controlling their thoughts, or plotting to harm them. These symptoms may leave them fearful and withdrawn. Their speech and behaviour can be so disorganised that they may be incomprehensible or frightening to others.

The combination of severe symptoms and chronic course of illness can cause a high degree of disability for those who suffer from schizophrenia.

Schizophrenia develops in about 1 in 100 people and can occur in men and women. Although schizophrenia affects men and women with equal frequency, the disorder often appears earlier in men. Men are usually affected in their late teens or early twenties, while women are generally affected in their twenties to early thirties.

Researchers are not sure what causes schizophrenia. However, problems with brain structure and chemistry are thought to play a role. There also appears to be a genetic component. Some theories propose that a viral infection in infancy and/or severe first trimester stress may increase the risk of schizophrenia in people who are predisposed.

Schizophrenia can also increase a person's risk of suicide, self-mutilation, substance abuse, and other social problems, such as being unemployed, homeless, and incarcerated. Obsessive-Compulsive Disorder (OCD) affects a significant number of people with schizophrenia.

The symptoms of schizophrenia fall into three broad categories: **positive** symptoms, **negative** symptoms, and **cognitive** symptoms.

Positive Symptoms

Positive symptoms are psychotic behaviours not seen in healthy individuals. People with positive symptoms often "lose touch" with reality and the symptoms can come and go. Sometimes they are severe and at other times hardly noticeable, and include the following:

Hallucinations are things a person sees, hears, smells, or feels that no one else can see, hear, smell, or feel. "Voices" are the most common type of hallucination in schizophrenia; many people with the disorder hear voices. The voices may talk to the person about his/her behaviour and sometimes order the person to do things, or warn the person of danger. Some people experience the voices talking to each other.

It's not unusual for people with schizophrenia to hear voices for a long time before family and friends notice the problem.

Other types of hallucinations include seeing people or objects that are not there, smelling odours that no one else detects, and feeling things like invisible fingers touching their bodies when no one is near.

Delusions are false beliefs that are not part of the person's culture and do not change (fixed beliefs); the person believes in the delusions even after other people prove that the beliefs are not true or logical. People with schizophrenia can have delusions that seem bizarre, such as believing that neighbours can control their behaviour with magnetic waves. They may also believe that people on television are directing special messages to them, or that radio stations are broadcasting their thoughts aloud to others. Sometimes they believe they are someone else, such as a famous historical figure. They may have paranoid delusions and believe that others are trying to harm them, such as by cheating, harassing, poisoning, spying on, or plotting against them or the people they care about. These beliefs are called "delusions of persecution."

Thought disorders are unusual or dysfunctional ways of thinking. One form of thought disorder is called "disorganised thinking." This is when a person has trouble organising his or her thoughts or connecting them logically. They may talk in a garbled way that is hard to understand. Another form is called "thought blocking." This is when a person stops speaking abruptly in the middle of a thought. When asked why he or she stopped talking, the person may say that it felt as if the thought had been taken out of his or her head. Finally, a person with a thought disorder might make up meaningless words, or newly coined words "neologisms."

Movement disorders may appear as agitated body movements. A person with a movement disorder may repeat certain motions over and over. In the other extreme, a person may become catatonic. Catatonia is a state in which a person does not move and does not respond to others. Catatonia is rare today, but it was more common when treatment for schizophrenia was not available.

<u>Negative Symptoms</u>

Negative symptoms are associated with disruptions to normal emotions and behaviours. These symptoms are harder to recognise as part of the disorder and can be mistaken for depression or other conditions. These symptoms include the following:

- "Flat affect" (a person's face does not move or he/she talks in a dull or monotonous voice)
- Lack of pleasure in everyday life
- Lack of ability to begin and sustain planned activities
- Speaking little, even when forced to interact.

People with negative symptoms need help with everyday tasks. They often neglect basic personal hygiene. This may make them seem lazy or unwilling to help themselves, but the problems are symptoms caused by the Schizophrenia.

Cognitive Symptoms

Cognitive symptoms are subtle. Like negative symptoms, cognitive symptoms may be difficult to recognise as part of the disorder. Often, they are detected only when other tests are performed. Cognitive symptoms include the following:

- Poor "executive functioning" (the ability to understand information and use it to make decisions)

- Trouble focusing or paying attention

- Problems with "working memory" (the ability to use information immediately after learning it).

Cognitive symptoms often make it hard to lead a normal life and earn a living. They can cause great emotional distress.

Nutritional Supplementation and Schizophrenia

(Pataracchia, 2002).

Be aware that nutritional supplementation and dietary interventions for serious mental illnesses is best done under supervision of a trained professional, such as a Clinical Nutritionist.

Nutritional needs of people with schizophrenia ultimately involve neurotransmitter issues of production, release, inhibition, transmission, and receptor formation. In schizophrenia, nutrition must also address neuron cell degeneration – an unfortunate, common finding in chronic schizophrenia. Neurotransmitter metabolism is intricately involved with chemical reactions which are in turn dependent on vitamins, minerals, and other substances. When diet cannot provide these missing nutritional substances, additional nutrient supplements become a necessity.

People with schizophrenia have peculiar nutritional profiles. Schizophrenia may be caused by genetic predisposing factors or environmental influences.

The nutritional approaches for schizophrenia highlighted in this book are as described by Dr. Abram Hoffer M.D. N.D. and Dr. Carl C. Pfeiffer M.D. (now deceased). The methods reflect the principles of evidence-based medicine.

Prognostic outcomes for these practitioners/researchers are as follows:

Abram Hoffer:

Period of sickness	with nutritional treatment lasting	becoming well & much improved
1 year (or in 2nd or 3rd relapse)	Up to 1 year	90% of patients
2-5 years	Up to 5 years	75% of patients
More than 5 years and out of mental hospital	5 or more years	50% of patients
More than 5 years and in a mental hospital	5 or more years	25% of patients

Carl Pfeiffer:

In the 1970's, Dr. Pfeiffer reported B_6 and zinc supplementation as being 95% successful in the management of over 400 cases of Pyroluria-type Schizophrenia. He also reported that lab-based orthomolecular nutritional protocols that alter neurotransmitter production can take 1 week to 1 year to take effect before symptoms start alleviating.

William J. Walsh, from the Pfeiffer Treatment Centre (P.T.C.), reports: low histamine schizophrenic patients experience, "major improvement within 6 weeks, but a year of treatment is commonly required before the last symptom (usually paranoia) can be overcome". High histamine treatment, "requires great patience, because six to ten weeks are often needed before the beginning of significant improvement."

These patients have depressive symptoms that begin to lift somewhere between 1-3 months; blank-mindedness symptoms that start leaving after 4-6 weeks but sometimes only after 4 months; obsessive symptoms that take somewhere between 3-6 weeks; compulsive symptoms that take 6-12 weeks; and phobic symptoms that take sometimes 1 year to dispel.

Most schizophrenic patients, according to referring psychiatrists, improve significantly following nutritional treatment, have fewer side effects from drugs, and are able to use lower doses of medications. Complete freedom from medications is not always possible for those with severe mental debilities.

An outcome study of 150 schizophrenic patients from the P.T.C. reports best results for patients under the age of 40.

The prognostic outcomes above are derived from patients who maintained regular medications until their biochemistry was balanced and remained stable for a couple of months, after which time regular medications were reduced (slowly) until none or very little medication was required.

Intervening with nutrition in the early stages improves the prognosis. Brain chemistry can be re-aligned more easily before this disease compromises brain cell structure. Therefore, the importance of early intervention cannot be over-emphasised.

Brain cell integrity must be addressed to avoid regression of brain tissue. This is important because damaged brain cells cannot be repaired. Essential fatty acid studies (described below and in many sections of this book, including the appendix section) have produced supportive evidence for their role in keeping neuron degeneration at bay and reducing psychotic symptoms.

Association between Schizophrenia and Omega 3: What's the Evidence?

(See also Appendix C: *Schizophrenia and Nutritional Studies*)

EFA's, including omega-3 and omega-6, are good fats, not saturated with hydrogen, and, unfortunately, not readily provided in the Western diet. 60 % of the dry weight of the brain is fat. William Walsh reports an integral need for appropriate EFA supplementation in schizophrenia, ADHD, and depression.

EFA's are important components of nerve cell walls and are involved in neurotransmitter electrical activity and post-receptor phospholipid-mediated signal transduction. Neuronal degeneration is found commonly among people with chronic schizophrenia as they have apparent increased phospholipid neuron membrane breakdown which concentrates in the frontal cortex and other areas of the brain.

EFA's offer a means of maintaining brain membrane structure and avoiding brain mass loss. Some specific EFA supplements are useful in schizophrenia and help to keep neuron degeneration at bay.

The likely course of schizophrenia is improved with custom vitamin-mineral supplementation because it is easier to take these supplements, and the ingredients are of higher quality than over the counter forms. Over the counter forms tend to have added ingredients that, in many cases, are contradictory to the supplement prescription.

Randomized, Placebo-Controlled Study of Ethyl-Eicosapentaenoic Acid as Supplemental Treatment in Schizophrenia.
(Emsley, Myburgh, Oosthuizen, & van Rensburg, 2002)

Abstract:

CONCLUSIONS: EPA may be an effective and well-tolerated add-on treatment in Schizophrenia.

Omega-3 polyunsaturated fatty acids may offer an

affordable treatment alternative. Supportive findings include low levels of omega-3 polyunsaturated fatty acids in red blood cells and the brain in Schizophrenia. Open-label supplemental studies have suggested a beneficial effect for omega-3 polyunsaturated fatty acids in Schizophrenia.

A pilot study found that eicosapentaenoic acid (EPA) was superior to docohexaenoic acid and placebo when added to standard antipsychotic treatment, although another double-blind study of EPA versus placebo found no improvement of symptoms with EPA.

In a dose-ranging study, ethyl-EPA (E-EPA) doses of 1, 2, and 4 g/day were no better than placebo, although subjects taking Clozapine with E-EPA improved significantly, the effect being greatest with a 2 g/day dose of E-EPA.

Recent reviews of the treatment of schizophrenia with omega-3 polyunsaturated fatty acids found results to be encouraging but preliminary, somewhat conflicting, and requiring independent replication.

Cerebral/Brain Allergies

10%-15% of people with schizophrenia have cerebral/brain allergies. Cerebral allergies involve a gut reaction that ultimately perpetuates the release of brain toxins, resulting in psychosis, malaise, etc (see also

Appendix E: *Bacteria & the Brain: The Powerful Behaviour Modifying Effects of the Gut)*.

Culprit foods and culprit environmental compounds have been identified in schizophrenia. An investigative procedure called "elimination dieting" is important for diagnosis. Individualised nutritional guidelines, assessment and patient histories can provide comprehensive programs of diet that can be essential in the management of schizophrenia. Testing for overpopulated gut micro-organisms such as Candida albicans is a vital part of the assessment when cerebral allergies are suspected. Mal-absorption also has to be ruled out.

<u>Sugar Imbalance</u>

Hypoglycaemia is the term that describes low sugar in the blood. Irritability, poor memory, "late afternoon blues", poor concentration, tiredness, cold hands, muscle cramping, and "feeling better when fighting" are typical hypoglycemic symptoms. Hypoglycaemia tends to be an aggravating factor in mental illnesses rather than a causative factor.

The nutritional protocol for hypoglycaemia involves dietary changes and supplemental support. It is said that hypoglycaemia is 100% treatable in compliant patients, emphasizing the need to adhere to the diet.

Vitamin B$_3$ Dependency

Niacin or niacinamide or niacin hexaniacinate are different forms of vitamin B$_3$. Vitamin B$_3$ can limit the conversion of norepinephrine to epinephrine (adrenaline). Excess adrenaline or excess catecholamines such as dopamine (implicated in the dopamine hypothesis of schizophrenia) are problematic as they can oxidise and form endogenous toxins.

The brain, with similar local reactions, may fail to store excess catecholamines – a job normally reserved for neuromelanin, hence allowing free circulation of neurotoxins. B$_3$ dependent pathways in the body vent the biochemistry of the body away from the formation of oxidised catecholamines and toxic indoles. This might under certain circumstances contribute to synaptic deletion. Abnormalities in this neuromelanin storage pathway may be considered causative factors in schizophrenia or Parkinson's disease. This biochemical theory was the first presented in medical literature by Dr. Hoffer and Dr. Humphry Osmond. This theory is called the adrenochrome hypothesis.

Niacin also plays a role in the essential fatty acid metabolism of the brain, processes of which are disrupted in schizophrenia. Niacin and vitamin C (ascorbic acid) are centrally active in the brain; "niacinamide in the brain acts on the diazepine receptors, while ascorbic acid acts on the dopamine receptors – as do Haldol and other [neuroleptics or] tranquilisers," (Dr. Hoffer).

The nutritional need/dependency versus deficiency (a less dependent state) for B_3 may indeed exceed the need to address any other nutritional metabolic compromise, as it is perhaps ultimately involved in the metabolism of the mind in people with schizophrenia.

Dr. Hoffer and Dr. Osmond spearheaded this nutritional approach, which includes appropriate sufficient doses of niacin. Other nutrients which complement 'niacin therapy', or the B_3 approach, have been clinically tested in several double-blind placebo-controlled trials, and overall assessment of these sources reveals sufficient evidence in support of B_3 therapy in the management of schizophrenia.

The six double-blinds done by Hoffer et al. were the first double-blind placebo-controlled trials ever done in the history of psychiatry. The B_3 therapy is discussed in detail in various journals and sources which include effectiveness and proposed mechanisms of action.

Dr. Abram Hoffer M.D. N.D. successfully treated over 4000 patients with this approach.

<u>Histamine Metabolism</u>

Carl Pfeiffer studied more than 20,000 people with schizophrenia, and determined that 90% of them fell into three bio-chemical subgroups: high histamine, low histamine, and Pyroluria - hence the term "The Schizophrenias".

Histamine is a reflection of neurotransmitter availability. Histamine is integral in balancing the electrical activity of the nucleus accumbens, which is an area of the brain responsible for behavioural responses, filtering incoming sensory information and communicating with the hypothalamus, ventral tegmentum, and amygdala.

An abundance of research has determined that people with schizophrenia have poor ability to filter incoming sensory information. It has also been reported that 15-20 % of people with schizophrenia have high whole blood histamine levels and another 30-40% of people with schizophrenia have low whole blood histamine levels.

A person with schizophrenia who has high histamine is under-methylated and a person with schizophrenia who has low histamine is over-methylated. Taking detailed patient histories is vital. People with high histamine have been found with typical symptoms of high intelligence, thought blanking, low grade hallucinations and thought disorder, perfectionism, competitiveness, obsessions, compulsions, suicidal and seasonal depression, defiance, and phobia.

High histamine individuals are inherently high in folic acid. Although folic acid is used along with B_{12} in the production of methionine it is also involved in histamine production along with B_{12}. Consequently B_{12} and folic acid are strictly avoided in high histamine patient care. These patients need to avoid multi-vitamins.

People with low histamine have been found with typical symptoms of under-achievement, more severe thought disorder and hallucinations, paranoid thoughts with less pronounced obsessions, suicidal depression, cyclic or suicidal depression, and anxiety.

Pyroluria Disorder

According to Dr. Pfeiffer, 30-50 % of people with schizophrenia have Pyroluria. Dr. Hoffer claimed that perhaps 70% of acute schizophrenia cases have Pyroluria, and that recovered patients have no Pyroluria.

What is Pyroluria and how is this related to brain function?

In some people, one specific Pyroluria – 2,4 dimethyl-3-ethylpyrrole – is produced in excess and excreted in the urine. 2,4 dimethyl-3-ethylpyrrole interacts with B_6, zinc and magnesium, leaving these nutrients deficient.

Pyroluria disorder individuals have problems forming serotonin, dopamine, GABA, norepinephrine, and glycine. B_6 is needed for proper brain detoxification. Zinc is essential in nerve development, intellectual function, serotonin formation, the regulation of mood, and the prevention of oxidative damage.

Pyroluria disorder is a condition of the whole body with both physical and mental symptoms, versus other nutritional bio-types of schizophrenia where there exists a typical resiliency to physical disease. Pyroluria disorder is common in behaviour disorders as well.

Specific behaviours and physical symptoms are associated with Pyroluria. People with Pyroluria-type schizophrenia may have classic delusions, classic hallucinations, lethargy, high internal tension, stress intolerance, assaultive behaviour, and unconstrained irritability. They may experience a single convulsion on administration of neuroleptics – when first prescribed. They tend to have more intact insight and better mood regulation than other nutritional biotypes but their social withdrawal seems more prominent.

Physical symptoms of knee joint pain and fingernail white spots are also common in Pyroluria. Dr. Pfeiffer and BioCentre Laboratory records from Wichita, Kansas, have noted an approximately 20% incidence of fingernail white spots and knee joint pain in people with schizophrenia. They tend to be female and sometimes have a "China doll", unhealthy, pale appearance (see also Appendix D: *An Interview: Dr. Bonnet Discusses Pyroluria*).

More and more research is highlighting the links between mental disorders and physical health problems. Schizophrenia, for example, is often shown to have links to the risk of developing other diseases and disorders, which can be physical or mental. The following chapters will highlight some of the impact of issues related to mental and physical health co-morbidity.

THE BODY IS a whole system; your brain is part of your body and one part cannot function optimally without the other. It's about balance. The bodily organs are made up of cells, and the organs of the body together make up the human being – the system. To survive we know that we need to be eating nourishing foods, to feed the cells of the body.

It is known that whenever a person is suffering from a prolonged mental illness they end up with many physical illnesses as well, and vice-versa. If a person has heart problems often they'll suffer depression and other kinds of mental health problems as well.

This co-morbidity demonstrates the urgency of taking collaboration – between service providers and service users – to the next level. To include survivor-led services, so that people don't get stuck in the system and become institutionalised; remaining on high levels of medication long-term without any option of moving away from that and getting well.

After such a prolonged period of medication, the brain-chemistry actually becomes altered and then there are issues with co-morbidity and lifespan. So, you can't just look at mental health in isolation, ignoring physical health.

Co-Morbidity of Mental and Physical Health Problems

Mental and physical health are both inextricably co-morbid.

Co-morbidity is the occurrence of more than one condition/disorder at the same time, and is common among those with mental illness. It can involve more than one mental disorder, or one mental disorder and one or more physical conditions. People with multiple disorders are more disabled and consume more health resources than those with only one disorder.

"The time is right to explore how patients with combined mental and physical health needs can be supported in a more integrated way."
(Naylor, et al., 2012)

The presence of a greater number of physical health problems is reported to contribute to more severe psychosis and depression. People with serious mental illness , such as schizophrenia and mood disorders, have higher rates of physical illness than the general population. Conversely, people with chronic physical health conditions experience depression and anxiety.

Co-existing mental and physical conditions can diminish quality of life and lead to longer illness duration and worse health outcomes.

This situation also generates economic costs to society due to increased heath service use and lost work productivity.

Understanding the links between mind and body is the first step in developing strategies to reduce the incidence of co-existing conditions and support those already living with mental and chronic physical illness.

According to Sean Duggan (Chief Executive at the Centre for Mental Health), it's, "Time to tackle the artificial divide between physical and mental health... improving the management of co-morbidity should not just be an add-on, but the norm in the provision of both physical and mental health care. An artificial divide between physical and mental health is no longer tenable in an NHS that values quality, integration and value for money. Understanding both, and the way they interact, is... fundamental to 21st century health care practice," (Naylor, et al., 2012).

Key points from the King's Fund report:

• Many people with long-term physical health conditions also have mental health problems. These can lead to significantly poorer health outcomes and reduced quality of life.

• Costs to the health care system are also significant – by interacting with and exacerbating physical illness, co-morbid mental health problems raise total health care costs by at least 45 per cent for each person with a long-term condition and co-morbid mental health problem.

• This suggests that between 12 per cent and 18 per cent of all NHS expenditure on long-term conditions is linked to poor mental health and wellbeing – between £8 billion and £13 billion in England each year. The more conservative of these figures equates to around £1 in every £8 spent on long-term conditions.

• People with long-term conditions and co-morbid mental health problems disproportionately live in deprived areas and have access to fewer resources of all kinds. The interaction between co-morbidities and deprivation makes a significant contribution to generating and maintaining inequalities.

• Care for large numbers of people with long-term conditions could be improved by better integrating mental health support with primary care and chronic disease management programmes, with closer working between mental health specialists and other professionals.

• Collaborative care arrangements between primary care and mental health specialists can improve outcomes with no or limited additional net costs.

• Innovative forms of liaison psychiatry demonstrate that providing better support for co-morbid mental health needs can reduce physical health care costs in acute hospitals.

• Clinical commissioning groups should prioritise integrating mental and physical health care more closely as a key part of their strategies to improve quality and productivity in health care.

• Improved support for the emotional, behavioural and mental health aspects of physical illness could play an important role in helping the NHS to meet the Quality, Innovation, Productivity and Prevention (QIPP) challenge. This will require removal of policy barriers to integration, for example, through redesign of payment mechanisms.

• Mental health problems are the largest single source of disability in the United Kingdom, accounting for 23% of the total 'burden of disease' (Department of Health).

• Between £8 billion and £13 billion of NHS spending in England is attributed to co-morbid mental health problems among people with long-term conditions (Depart of Health figures 2010).

It's not uncommon to find that disturbed sleep patterns are key symptoms of many psychiatric disorders. When these sleep disturbances are properly addressed, significant improvement in psychiatric symptoms can result. In the following chapter we'll be looking at some of the associations between mental disorders and sleep.

THE PROBLEM CAME when I stopped sleeping. I didn't feel that I needed to sleep, but the lack of sleep caused me to experience different delusions and hallucinations. I got to a point where I started to see and hear things that weren't there, to have strange beliefs about myself and other people, paranoia started to set in and I believed that I knew what other people were thinking and vice-versa.

Things were spiralling so far out of control that I began to experience a sensation of travelling through time, as though I was awake but asleep at the same time. It was like being in a Twilight Zone where I was unable to distinguish reality from delusion. I had so much energy, and I felt I had a direct connection with God. At the same time I didn't have a concept of what God was supposed to be, so that anyone and anything could be God. I began preaching in the streets and was eventually taken to hospital and placed on a section.

I have since learned the importance of sleep. Sleep helps the body to repair and replenish; it helps the body to rebalance itself. I paid attention, not just to the act of sleeping, but to the type of sleep I was getting – I wanted quality sleep. I learned that certain nutrients would produce the hormones that bring about quality sleep. This is where, again, the link with diet comes in – there's no getting away from it.

Circadian Clock: A Timing System in the Suprachiasmatic Nuclei (SCN) of the Hypothalamic Region of the Brain

Circadian rhythms are rhythms in our body that alternate about every 24 hours. 'Circa' means 'about', 'dian' means 'day' so circadian rhythms have what's called a period of about 24 hours.

This internal clock system is composed of an intracellular feedback loop that drives the expression of molecular components and their constitutive protein products to oscillate over a period of about 24 hours (hence the term 'circadian'). These circadian oscillations bring about rhythmic changes in downstream molecular pathways and physiological processes such as those involved in nutrition and metabolism.

It is now emerging that the molecular components of the clock system are also found within the cells of peripheral tissues, including the gastrointestinal tract, liver and pancreas. The present review examines their role in regulating nutritional and metabolic processes. In turn, metabolic status and feeding cycles are able to feed back onto the circadian clock in the SCN and in peripheral tissues. This feedback mechanism maintains the integrity and temporal coordination between various components of the circadian clock system. Thus, alterations in environmental cues could disrupt normal clock function, which may have profound effects on the health and well-being of an individual (Cagampang & Bruce, 2012).

Circadian rhythms are physical, mental and behavioural changes that follow a roughly 24-hour cycle, responding primarily to light and darkness in an organism's environment. They are found in most living things, including animals, plants and many tiny microbes. The study of circadian rhythms is called chronobiology (National Institute of General Medical Sciences, 2012)

Sleep and Disruption of Circadian Rhythms

Sleep is an important part of our daily lives. It helps restore our energy, keep our memory functioning properly, and helps to heal our bodies. When sleep is disrupted or deprived, we don't feel as alert as we could, we are easily agitated and all of our actions seem slow and drawn out. It is common that stress and anxiety from demands of work, family, and everyday life lead to sleeping problems.

As time has passed, people's lives have become much faster paced. From hectic work schedules, travelling and much more involvement in social activities, we leave little time for ourselves to unwind and relax. Because our lives have been significantly sped up, we tend to get less sleep causing many of us to feel run down and exhausted.

Natural Rhythm of Mind and Body

Many of the rhythms of our body and mind are synchronised with nature. For example, when our biological clock is functioning properly, the wake drive will start to increase in the morning, as the sun is rising. The circadian system and the sleep-wake system then prompts our bodies to produce cortisol, serotonin, and other hormones that wake us up, increase blood pressure and cause body temperature to rise. Likewise, at sunset, the body receives another cue and responds to the lack of sunlight by producing and releasing the hormone melatonin. Unlike at sunrise, this leads to a decrease in blood pressure and allows the body to prepare for and eventually fall into sleep.

So, when our bodies are out of sync with the 24-hour Circadian rhythm cycle, rhythm is not regular, and hormone and neurotransmitter release is negatively affected, causing our bodies to potentially suffer from a circadian rhythm disorder (CRD), influencing depression.

Can Our Eating and Drug Habits Affect Circadian Rhythm?

The circadian clock is strongly influenced by diet: in fact, food intake dominates light in setting the circadian clock. If you regularly eat at night and fast during the day, the body will start treating night as day and day as night (Fuller, Lu, & Saper, 2008).

When it comes to addiction, research has shown that people with circadian rhythm disruption are more vulnerable to addiction. Drugs of abuse can entrain circadian rhythms, such that drug use is anticipated by the brain, leading to increased craving and drug seeking behaviour.

So, for example, if you get into the habit of having an alcoholic drink in the evening at 5 o'clock, your brain reward system will start to anticipate those drinks at 5 o'clock. And at about 4-4:30, you might start thinking about those drinks, wanting them and craving them. It's because the reward system has been set by that drug.

Also long-term exposure to drugs of abuse leads to disruptions in the circadian system, causing long lasting mood and sleep problems.

Additionally, an important point to note is that circadian rhythm disruption can also suppress immune function which increases vulnerability to infectious disease.

Our Biological Clocks Drive our Circadian Rhythms.

The biological clocks that control circadian rhythms are groupings of interacting molecules in cells throughout the body. A "master clock" in the brain coordinates all the body clocks so that they are in sync.

The "master clock" that controls circadian rhythms consists of a group of nerve cells in the brain called the suprachiasmatic nucleus, or SCN. The SCN contains about 20,000 nerve cells and is located in the hypothalamus, an area of the brain just above where the optic nerves from the eyes cross.

Researchers have already identified genes that direct circadian rhythms in people, fruit flies, mice, fungi and several other model organisms used for studying genetics.

Circadian rhythms are produced by natural factors within the body, but they are also affected by signals from the environment. Light is the main cue influencing circadian rhythms, turning on or turning off genes that control an organism's internal clock.

Circadian rhythms can influence sleep-wake cycles, hormone release, body temperature and other important bodily functions. They have been linked to various sleep disorders, such as insomnia. Abnormal circadian rhythms have also been associated with obesity, diabetes, depression, bipolar disorder, schizophrenia and seasonal affective disorder.

Circadian rhythms are important in determining human sleep patterns. The body's master clock, or SCN, controls the production of melatonin, a hormone that makes you sleepy. Since it is located just above the optic nerves, which relay information from the eyes to the brain, the SCN receives information about incoming light. When there is less light – like at night – the SCN tells the brain to make more melatonin so you get drowsy.

Circadian Rhythm Disorders

A circadian rhythm disorder (CRD) means your body is producing hormones, chemicals and neurotransmitters in the wrong amounts and/or at the wrong time of the day. The timing of psychological, behavioural, physiological, and hormonal rhythms with respect to the day-night cycle, clearly displays how regular patterns and chronological order are essential for optimal health.

Consequently, when our bodies are not in tune with nature's biological cues, this has the potential to lead to negative effects on our mental and physical wellbeing. Because circadian rhythms control the release and timing of hormones, CRD underlies many mood disorders and sleep disruption.

The Role of Melatonin

Melatonin is an important night-time hormone associated with sleep and regeneration. However, excessive levels can cause depressive disorders. This hormone is normally released at night as the sunlight disappears, causing people to become tired. If we are awake with melatonin in our system we often exhibit some of the following symptoms: lethargy, disorientation, irritability and moodiness. This explains why depression is highest in the darkest climates. Almost everyone with a mood disorder suffers the most in the winter because of the excessive melatonin in our system. Some of the Seasonal Affective Disorder effects may also be due to a lack of light exposure, which can affect melatonin secretion, circadian timing (inducing phase shifts) and also has direct alerting effects.

Depression and Seasonal Affective Disorder (SAD)

People suffering from depression may have a malfunction in their biological clock, resulting in skewed hormone release. Our body needs serotonin to be active and energetic during the day and melatonin to help pull us back to sleep. But, if the brain is triggered to secrete melatonin during the day, it can cause us to feel dull, unstable, irritable and moody. Oftentimes depression is the result of our bodies producing the wrong hormones at the wrong time of day. This imbalance in the circadian system can be caused from lack of sleep, stress, trauma, inappropriate timing of sleep-wake periods, genetic factors, shift-work, or lack of light.

SAD is the most closely related disorder to CRD. During the months of the year when the days become shorter, the brain's master clock receives insufficient amounts of light, causing it to miss certain cues to release necessary chemicals. This can cause malfunctions and result in the production of the wrong hormones at the wrong time of day.

Research also shows that without sunlight, the brain doesn't produce enough serotonin, resulting in the symptoms of depression. The darker days also signal the brain to overproduce melatonin. The symptoms diminish as the days get longer, although many SAD sufferers note brief (1-2 week) periods of SAD like symptoms in the summer (Mental Health Wiki, 2010).

Circadian Cycle and Bipolar Disorder

For a long time there has been interest in the question of whether problems in the circadian cycle, or the sleep-wake cycle has something to do with what causes bipolar disorder.

A number of studies have shown that when people are manic or when they are depressed they have trouble with their sleep-wake cycle. When they are manic they don't sleep and they don't really care about sleeping; they aren't tired. When they are depressed, typically they want to sleep a lot. This makes evident that these problems are symptoms... but does it prove that the problems are indeed related to the sleep-wake cycle?

Evidence from studies has emerged showing that if you take someone who has bipolar disorder and you keep them awake for all or part of the night, they have a rather significant chance of becoming manic. So researchers have concluded that such disturbances in the sleep-wake cycle can actually cause problems in the mood cycle.

Moreover, what these studies have demonstrated is that you can drive the mood cycle by disturbing the sleep wake cycle. That's very important clinically, because in some of the treatments for bipolar disorder, what they try to do is to stabilise the sleep-wake cycle.

What becomes clear is that people with bipolar disorder should try to stay on a pretty regular sleep-wake cycle. For example, people with bipolar disorder may have a great deal of difficulty with shift work or with jet lag, they may have mood shifts when they suffer jet lag.

Bipolar sufferers may also experience that sleep problems feel worse at a particular time of day. Because these symptoms reflect a CRD, doctors have found some success by treating bipolar disorders with bright light.

Light Therapy and Depression

Researchers have discovered how exposure to bright light stimulates the production of brain chemicals to relieve symptoms related to depressive disorders. Light exposure suppresses melatonin and helps to reset the internal biological clock.

The circadian system gains information about the time of day from the environment via various time cues, with the strongest being changes in light-dark exposure. The circadian system is sensitive to 'normal' light exposure, with specialised receptors in the eye, not used for vision, being stimulated by light entering the eye and information transported to the hypothalamus. It has recently been discovered that these circadian specialised receptors in the eye are more sensitive to particular wavelengths of light or blue light.

When a person is exposed to light, it enters the eye via the optic nerve and activates the hypothalamus. Once triggered, the hypothalamus sends a signal to the pineal gland which immediately suppresses the production of melatonin and stimulates the production of serotonin. When serotonin is released, negative symptoms are alleviated, making you feel alert and active.

Light therapy can be used as a treatment for sleep disorders as well as to reduce the duration of jetlag, by increasing the rate of circadian adaptation as well as via a direct alerting effect.

It has been found that by using blue light for light therapy, the time of exposure to the light may be shortened, and the brightness of the light may be reduced compared to when 'normal' lights with all different wavelengths included are used.

Circadian Rhythm Disruption in Schizophrenia

Sleep and circadian rhythm disruption (SCRD) and schizophrenia are often co-morbid.

Recent clinical evidence supports that the treatment of SCRD leads to improvements in both the sleep quality and psychiatric symptoms of schizophrenia patients. Moreover, many SCRD-associated pathologies, such as impaired cognitive performance, are routinely observed in schizophrenia.

The relationship between schizophrenia and abnormal sleep was first described in the late nineteenth century by the German psychiatrist Emil Kraepelin (Manoach & Stickgold, 2009).

Today, sleep and circadian rhythm disruption (SCRD) is reported in 30-80% of patients with schizophrenia, and is increasingly recognised as one of the most common features of the disorder (Cohrs, 2008).

Sleep disturbances in schizophrenia include increases in sleep latency, and reductions in total sleep time, sleep efficiency, REM sleep latency, REM sleep density and slow-wave sleep duration (Cohrs, 2008); (Manoach & Stickgold, 2009).

Schizophrenia is also associated with significant circadian disruption, including the abnormal phasing, instability and fragmentation of rest-activity rhythms (Martin, et al., 2001), (2005); (Wulff, Joyce, Middleton, Dijk, & Foster, 2006); (Wulff, Porcheret, Cussans, & Foster, 2009).

Crucially, patients with SCRD score badly on many quality-of-life clinical subscales, highlighting the human cost of SCRD in schizophrenia (Cohrs, 2008); (Goldman, et al., 1996); (Hofstetter, Lysaker, & Mayeda, 2005). To reinforce this, schizophrenia patients often comment that an improvement in sleep is one of their highest priorities during treatment (Auslander & Jeste, 2002).

Clinical Evidence for Common Brain Mechanisms in SCRD and Schizophrenia

Sleep and circadian rhythm disruption is rarely targeted for treatment in schizophrenia, but when it is, patients report improvements in both their sleep quality and psychiatric symptoms (Kantrowitz, et al., 2010).

In a recent study, insomnia was treated in 15 patients with persistent persecutory delusions and schizophrenia (Myers, Startup, & Freeman, 2011). Following a cognitive behavioural therapy (CBT) intervention, there were significant reductions in both insomnia and persecutory delusions. At least two-thirds of participants showed a substantial improvement in insomnia, whilst approximately half showed a substantial reduction in persecutory delusions. There were also reductions in levels of hallucinations, anxiety and depression.

Although consistent with the existence of common mechanisms in SCRD and schizophrenia, the results of this study should be interpreted with caution, due to a number of methodological limitations; the sample size was small, there was no control group, and 14 of the 15 patients received antipsychotic medication during the CBT intervention.

Significantly, many of the pathologies caused by SCRD are routinely reported as co-morbid with schizophrenia, but are rarely linked to the disruption of sleep. For example, sleep deprivation (Alhola & Polo-Kantola, 2007); (Chee & Chuah, 2008); (Horne, 1993); (Van Dongen, Maislin, Mullington, & Dinges, 2003) and circadian de-synchronisation (Kyriacou & Hastings, 2010) are known to impair cognition in healthy individuals, and cognitive impairment is a core symptom of schizophrenia.

Thus, cognitive impairments in schizophrenia could be exacerbated by circadian de-synchronisation and/or disturbed sleep.

Consistent with this, associations between sleep and cognitive performance have been reported in medication-naïve (Forest, et al., 2007), medicated (Bromundt, et al., 2011); (Göder, et al., 2004), (2008); (Wulff & Joyce, 2011), and unmedicated schizophrenia patients (Yang & Winkelman, 2006). In the latter study, the severity of patients' cognitive symptoms was inversely related with slow-wave sleep duration and REM sleep density (Yang & Winkelman, 2006).

Memory impairment is prevalent in schizophrenia (Aleman, Hijman, de Haan, & Kahn, 1999), and it has been suggested that sleep makes a crucial contribution to memory consolidation (Stickgold, 2005). Reduced overnight consolidation of procedural learning has been demonstrated in schizophrenia patients (Manoach, et al., 2004), and more recently, this effect was linked to a reduction in slow-wave sleep duration (Manoach, et al., 2010). The negative symptoms of schizophrenia might also be sensitive to SCRD, since circadian de-synchronisation increases negative mood, irritability and affective volatility in healthy volunteers (Kyriacou & Hastings, 2010); (Murray & Harvey, 2010). Consistent with this, improvements in sleep quality are frequently correlated with the amelioration of negative symptoms in schizophrenia patients (Hofstetter, Lysaker, & Mayeda, 2005); (Yamashita, Mori, Okamoto, Morinobu, & Yamawaki, 2004).

"Mental health problems are the largest single source of disability in the United Kingdom, accounting for 23% of the total 'burden of disease'." (Naylor, et al., 2012).

Between £8 billion and £13 billion of NHS spending in England is attributed to co-morbid mental health problems among people with long-term conditions (Depart of Health figures, 2010).

Mental illness and Chronic Physical Conditions Co-Exist – Why?

Both mind and body are affected by changes to physiological and emotional processes, as well as factors such as diet choices, income and housing.

These pathways of biology, illness experience, and social determinants of health can increase the likelihood of someone living with a mental illness or chronic physical condition leading to a co-existing condition.

At a chemical level, the difference between mental and physical illness is almost indistinguishable.   The major difference between physical and mental illness is in the emergence of symptoms.

Both serious mental health illness and chronic physical illness are commonly disabling. These conditions can affect anyone, regardless of age, culture, race/ethnicity, gender or income status.

Generally, mental health care is provided by one part of the health sector, whilst physical health is provided by a different health sector. In some cases, one condition may be receiving adequate attention while the other is not. The consequence of fragmented or incomplete care is that the individual does not receive appropriate holistic care that looks at the "whole person", consequently these individuals may have a lower life expectancy and a poorer quality of life.

Mental and physical illnesses also share many symptoms, such as food cravings and decreased energy levels, which can increase food consumption, decrease physical activity and contribute to weight gain.

These factors increase the risk of developing chronic physical conditions and can also have a detrimental impact upon an individual's mental well-being.

Some chronic physical conditions can cause high blood sugar levels, disrupting the circulation of blood and impacting brain function.

The biological impact of high blood sugar levels is also associated with the development of depression in people with diabetes.

People living with chronic physical conditions often experience emotional stress and chronic pain, which are both associated with the development of depression and anxiety.

Experiences of disability can also cause distress and isolate people from social supports.

There is some evidence that the more symptomatic the chronic physical condition, the more likely that a person will also experience mental health problems. Thus, it is not surprising that people with chronic physical conditions often self-report poor mental health.

Furthermore, people with serious mental illness often experience high blood pressure and elevated levels of stress hormones and adrenaline, which increase the heart rate. Anti-psychotic medications have also been linked with the development of an abnormal heart rhythm.

These physical changes interfere with cardiovascular functioning and significantly elevate the risk of developing heart disease among people with mental illness. Similarly, people with serious mental illness also experience higher rates of many other risk factors for heart disease, such as poor nutrition (leading to obesity), lack of exercise, and lack of access to preventive health screenings. In addition to this, people with serious mental illnesses have up to a three times greater likelihood of having a stroke.

Conversely, there are significantly elevated rates of depression among people with heart disease. According to studies, it is three times more likely that a person with heart disease will experience depression, when compared to people who do not have heart problems. Depression also often occurs following a stroke.

Studies have also highlighted that people with serious mental illness have a significantly increased likelihood of developing a range of chronic respiratory conditions including Chronic Obstructive Pulmonary Disease (COPD), chronic bronchitis and asthma.

Smoking is commonly identified as a risk factor for respiratory illnesses. People with mental illness are known to have high smoking rates, due in part to the historical acceptability of smoking in psychiatric institutions. People living with chronic respiratory diseases can experience significantly elevated rates of anxiety and depression.

A co-existing mental and physical health problem can lead to poor self-care practices.

Reports also show that people who experience asthma attacks have a greater likelihood of experiencing anxiety and panic disorders. In addition, some asthma medications have been demonstrated to alter mood.

Research linking cancer and mental illness has produced mixed results. A 2001 research found significantly higher rates of cancer among people with schizophrenia than expected (Lichtermann, Ekelund, Pukkala, Tanskanen, & Lönngvist, 2001).

As can be seen from the examples of connections between mental and physical health, if these co-existing conditions are left unaddressed, they can, collectively, contribute to the worsening of both mental and physical health.

WHAT DROVE ME to look at research to do with the heart was my religion. There are a number of Islamic teachings that mention the heart and it being able to remember and think, for example.

I came across some research that had been conducted by an institution called HeartMath. They were looking at conditions such as anxiety and other things to do with how the heart influences certain mental conditions, etc. They found that the heart did indeed have a memory, and furthermore that it was in control of the brain – sending messages to the brain for the brain to decode.

Heightened distress is of critical importance as a potential trigger of acute coronary syndromes and cardiac arrhythmias, particularly among vulnerable individuals. There is a growing interest in the pathomechanisms by which the central nervous system modulates cardiac autonomic control in various mental disorders, as well as potential links between emotional, cognitive and cardiac activity.

What becomes clear is that psychological states have a dramatic impact on heart rate variability (HRV), which is emerging as an objective measure of individual differences in regulated emotional responding, particularly as it relates to social processes and mental health. And as we know, stress is a common factor in disease co-morbidity, including a variety of mental disorders.

Links and Interactions between Brain and Heart

"Every whole has a relationship with and is a part of a greater whole, which is again part of something greater. In this context, nothing can be considered as separate."
(Bohm & Hiley, 1993).

The concept of the mind is of central importance for psychiatrists and psychologists. However, in many cultures throughout history, the heart has been considered the source of emotions, passion and wisdom. In the past, scientists emphasised the role of the brain in the head as being responsible for such experiences.

There is considerable observational evidence for a link between psychological distress and cardiovascular diseases, and other coronary risk factors. Because of the overlap between somatic symptoms in cardiac and vascular diseases with those in depression and anxiety, it remains unclear whether there is a causal relationship.

However, several biological factors are shared between heart disease and psychological diseases, which have encouraged investigators to assess whether the relationship is simply an epiphenomenon, causal in one or both directions, and to what degree the relationship is genetic.

More recently, studies have explored the physiological mechanisms by which the heart communicates with the brain, thereby influencing information processing, perceptions, emotions and health.

These studies revealed that the heart appeared to be sending meaningful messages to the brain that it not only understood, but also obeyed (Lacey & Lacey, 1978). These studies have also provided a scientific basis to explain how and why the heart affects mental clarity, creativity and emotional balance.

Physical and Mental Health Disorders – A Co-Existing Problem

Quite often, physical and mental health disorders go hand in hand. Research has shown that persons with severe or chronic physical illnesses often have a co-existing mental health problem. At the same time, persons with severe mental illnesses or substance abuse disorders have physical health problems that often remain undetected or untreated. This situation – combined with the reality that there is still stigma associated with mental illness and that most persons first seek help through their GP – has resulted in an emphasis on the need for better integration between mental and physical health care.

People with severe mental illness experience an excess of coronary heart disease (CHD), morbidity and mortality (Brown, 1997); (Phelan, Stradins, & Morrison, 2001). Mortality rates for cardiovascular disease in this group are increasing, and it is CHD, not suicide, that is the biggest killer (Hansen, Jacobsen, & Arnesen, 2001); (Lawrence, Holman, Jablensky, & Hobbs, 2003). This may be exacerbated by the metabolic and endocrine effects of antipsychotics, including weight gain (Blackburn, 2000) and impaired glucose homeostasis (Haddad, 2004).

Major depressive disorder is a risk factor in the development of incident coronary heart disease events in healthy patients and for adverse cardiovascular outcomes in patients with established heart disease. For people with heart disease, depression can increase the risk of an adverse cardiac event such as a heart attack or blood clots. For people who do not have heart disease, depression can also increase the risk of a heart attack and development of coronary artery disease.

Depression has been proven to be such a risk factor in cardiac disease that the American Heart Association (AHA) has recommended that all cardiac patients be screened for depression.

A Dutch Study, led by Elizabeth J. Martens of Tilburg University in the Netherlands, found that anxiety disorders may increase the risk of heart attack, stroke, heart failure and death in people with heart disease. The research included over 1,000 people with stable coronary heart disease who were assessed for anxiety disorder at the start of the study and then followed for an average of 5.6 years.

During that time, there were a total of 371 cardiovascular events (heart attacks or other incidents that may cause damage to the heart). The yearly rate of cardiovascular events was 9.6% among the 106 patients with generalised anxiety disorder and 6.6% among the other 909 patients. After adjusting for a number of factors -- such as other health problems, heart disease severity and medication use -- the researchers concluded that generalised anxiety disorder was associated with a 74% increased risk of cardiovascular events (World Federation for Mental Health).

BBC News August 2012: Mild mental illness 'raises risk of premature death'

People with mild mental illnesses such as anxiety or depression are more likely to die early, say researchers.

They looked at the premature deaths from conditions such as heart disease and cancer of 68,000 people in England.

The research suggested low level distress raised the risk by 16%, once lifestyle factors such as drinking and smoking were taken into account.

More serious problems increased it by 67%, the University College London and Edinburgh University team said.

The risk among those with severe mental health problems is already well documented. But researchers said the finding among those with milder cases - thought to be one in every four people - was concerning, as many would be undiagnosed.

The Wellcome Trust-funded study, published in the British Medical Journal, looked at data over 10 years and matched it to information on death certificates.

This is the largest study so far to show an association between psychological distress and death, according to scientists.

Lead author Dr Tom Russ said: "The fact that an increased risk of mortality was evident, even at low levels of psychological distress, should prompt research into whether treatment of these very common, minor symptoms can modify this increased risk of death."

Paul Jenkins, chief executive of the charity Rethink, said: "Sadly, these findings do not come as a surprise.

"While this study looks at depression and anxiety, people with severe mental illnesses such as bipolar disorder and schizophrenia die, on average, 20 years earlier than the rest of us. It's an absolute scandal.

"There is a huge lack of awareness amongst health professionals about the increased risk of physical illness for this group, which means people are dying needlessly every day... It is a scandal that this group of people die on average 20 years younger than the general population, mostly due to preventable physical conditions... Too often mental health professionals overlook the physical health needs of their patients... At the same time, busy professionals don't always monitor the side effects from antipsychotic medication properly... Many of our members say that they are not taken seriously by doctors when they raise concerns about their physical health."

(Selvadurai, 2012)

Heart Brain Communications

It has long been known that changes in emotions are accompanied by predictable changes in the heart rate, blood pressure, respiration and digestion. So, when we are aroused, the sympathetic division of the autonomic nervous system energises us for fight or flight, and in more quiet times, the parasympathetic component cools us down. In this view, it was assumed that the autonomic nervous system and the physiological responses moved in concert with the brain's response to a given stimulus (Rein, Atkinson, & McCraty, 1995).

However, over the past several decades, several lines of scientific evidence have established that the heart functions as a sensory organ and as a complex information encoding and processing centre.

Groundbreaking research in the relatively new field of neurocardiology has demonstrated that the heart has an extensive intrinsic nervous system that is sufficiently sophisticated to qualify as a "little brain" in its own right.

Pioneer neurocardiology researcher Dr. J. Andrew Armour first described the anatomical organisation and function of the heart brain in 1991 (Armour, 1991). The heart's complex circuitry, containing over 40,000 neurons, enables it to sense, regulate, and remember. Moreover, the heart brain can process information and make decisions about cardiac control independent of the central nervous system, evidenced by the ability of the heart to survive the temporary (and sometimes permanent) loss of nerve connections to the brain during a heart transplant. The existence of an intrinsic nervous system within the heart itself in fact allows it to survive in a new host without the help of the brain. (Armour, Neurocardiology: Anatomical and Functional Principles, 1994); (Armour & Kember, 2004).

This new area of research provides evidence that the heart communicates with the mind and body through an inherent nervous system that can influence perception, decision-making, and overall health. The heart is in constant communication with the body and brain using neurons, biochemicals, blood pressure waves and electricity, and has its own independent nervous system, and therefore the heart has a much greater impact on information processing, perceptions, emotions and health than was ever acknowledged in the past.

Researchers with the Institute of HeartMath and other entities have shown that the heart brain communicates with the brain via a number of pathways, and the brain in turn communicates with the heart. Between them they continually exchange critical information that influences how the body functions.

Traditionally, the study of communication pathways between the "head" and heart has been approached from a rather one-sided perspective, with scientists focusing primarily on the heart's responses to the brain's commands. However, it is becoming clear that communication between the heart and brain is actually a dynamic, ongoing, two-way dialogue, with each organ continually influencing the other's function.

According to research findings by the Institute Of HeartMath: The heart communicates to the brain in four major ways:

- **Neurologically** (through the transmission of nerve impulses)
- **Biologically** (via hormones and neurotransmitters)
- **Biophysically** (through pressure waves)
- **Energetically** (through electromagnetic field interactions).

"Communication along these conduits significantly affects the brain's activity." (Institute of HeartMath, 2001).

The heart is the most powerful generator of electromagnetic energy in the human body, producing the largest rhythmic electromagnetic field of any of the body's organs. The heart's electrical field is about 60 times greater in amplitude than the electrical activity generated by the brain. This field, measured in the form of an electrocardiogram (ECG), can be detected anywhere on the surface of the body. Furthermore, the magnetic field produced by the heart is more than 5,000 times greater in strength than the field generated by the brain, and can be detected a number of feet away from the body, in all directions, using SQUID-based magnetometers (McCraty, 2003).

The heart's nervous system contains around 40,000 neurons, called sensory neurites (Armour, 1991). Information from the heart - including feeling sensations - is sent to the brain through several afferents. These afferent nerve pathways enter the brain at the area of the medulla, and cascade up into the higher centres of the brain, where they may influence perception, decision making and other cognitive processes (Armour, 2004).

Normally, the heart communicates with the brain via nerve fibres running through the vagus nerve and the spinal column. In a heart transplant, these nerve connections do not reconnect for an extended period of time; in the meantime, the transplanted heart is able to function in its new host only through the capacity of its intact, intrinsic nervous system (Murphy, et al., 2000).

The heart brain senses hormonal, heart rate, and blood pressure signals, translates them into neurological impulses, and processes this information internally. It then sends the information to the central brain via afferent pathways in the vagus nerves and spinal column. When different hormones or neurotransmitters in the bloodstream are detected by the sensory neurites in the heart, the pattern in the afferent neural output sent to the brain is modified (Armour, 1994). In other words, in addition to its better-known functions, the heart is also a sensory centre that detects and transmits information about the biochemical content of the regional blood flow.

Research has also revealed that the heart communicates information to the brain and throughout the body via electromagnetic field interactions. It is proposed that this heart field acts as a carrier wave for information that provides a global synchronising signal for the entire body (McCraty, Bradley, & Tomasino, 2004-2005).

There is evidence that a subtle yet influential electromagnetic or 'energetic' communication system operates just below our conscious awareness. Energetic interactions possibly contribute to the 'magnetic' attractions or repulsions that occur between individuals, and also affect social relationships. It was also found that one person's brain waves can synchronise to another person's heart (McCraty, 2003).

Neurological signals originating in the heart have an important and widespread influence in regulating the function of organs and systems throughout the body. For example, it is now known that in addition to modulating the activity of the nervous and endocrine systems, input from the heart influences the activity of the digestive tract, urinary bladder, spleen, respiratory and lymph systems, and skeletal muscles (Chernigovskiy, 1967).

In more specific terms, cardiovascular afferent signals regulate efferent ANS outflow, (Grossman, Jannsen, & Vaitl, 1986), modulate pain perception (Randich & Gebhart, 1992) and hormone production (Drinkhill & Mary, 1989), and influence the activity of the locus coeruleus and that of the pyramidal tract cells in the motor cortex (Coleridge, Coleridge, & Rosenthal, 1976); (Svensson & Thorén, 1979).

Also, spinal cord excitability varies directly with the cardiac pulse, as does physiological tremor of normal skeletal muscles (Forster & Stone, 1976).

Beyond the key role of cardiac afferent signals in physiological regulation, the heart also bears significant influence on perceptual and cognitive functions via its input to higher brain centres.

The Heart and Amygdala

Research has shown that the heart's afferent neurological signals directly affect activity in the amygdala and associated nuclei, an important emotional processing centre in the brain. The amygdala is the key brain centre that coordinates behavioural, immunological, and neuroendocrine responses to environmental threats. It compares incoming emotional signals with stored emotional memories, and accordingly makes instantaneous decisions about the level of perceived threat. Due to its extensive connections to the limbic system, it is able to take over the neural pathways, activating the autonomic nervous system and emotional response before the higher brain centres receive the sensory information (Rein, Atkinson, & McCraty, 1995); (McCraty, Atkinson, Tiller, Rein, & Wakins, 1995).

Biochemical Interactions Between Heart and Brain

Another component of the heart-brain communication system was provided by researchers studying the hormonal system. The heart was reclassified as an endocrine gland when, in 1983, a hormone produced and released by the heart called atrial natriuretic factor (ANF) was isolated and nicknamed the "balance hormone". This hormone was found to play an important role in fluid and electrolyte homeostasis. It exerts its effect on the blood vessels, on the kidneys, the adrenal glands, and on a large number of regulatory regions in the brain. It was also found that the heart contains a cell type known as 'intrinsic cardiac adrenergic' (ICA) cells. These cells release noradrenaline and dopamine neurotransmitters, once thought to be produced only by neurons in the brain and ganglia outside of the heart (Huang, et al., 1996).

Dopamine and noradrenaline play important roles in high-level executive functions often reported to be impaired in attention-deficit/hyperactivity disorder (ADHD).

What is Noradrenaline?

The terms noradrenaline (from the Latin) and norepinephrine (derived from Greek) are interchangeable. It is known to increase heart rate and blood pressure. It is used to dilate pupils and air passages inside the lungs. Norepinephrine prevents narrowing of blood vessels in visceral organs. This allows the body to perform well in stressful situations and it stimulates a type of receptor known as adrenoceptors, which are scattered in all parts of the body.

The synthesis of norepinephrine begins with the synthesis of dopamine. Once dopamine is synthesised and stored in the synaptic vesicles, an enzyme called Dopamine β-hydroxylase (DBH) further hydroxylates dopamine into norepinephrine.

Functionally, the noradrenergic system can be viewed as a modulatory system because it can increase the "signal to noise ratio" of responses evoked by other neurotransmitters that excite or inhibit target cells (Woodward, Moises, Waterhouse, Yeh, & Cheun, 1991).

As a stress hormone, norepinephrine affects parts of the brain such as the amygdala, where attention and responses are controlled. Along with epinephrine, norepinephrine also underlies the fight-or-flight response, directly increasing heart rate, triggering the release of glucose from energy stores, and increasing blood flow to skeletal muscle. It also increases the brain's oxygen supply.

Almost every part of the brain receives input from noradrenergic neurons. These circuits are involved in controlling alertness, concentration and energy.

What is dopamine?

Dopamine is a neurotransmitter that plays a number of roles, including pleasurable reward, movement, memory and attention. It is thought to play a role in a number of diseases through its deficiency or excess. For example, Parkinson's disease and drug addiction are among the problems associated with abnormal dopamine levels.

Dopamine transmission in the pre frontal cortex (PFC) is directly involved in cognitive processes (Seamans & Yang, 2004), in the regulation of emotions (Sullivan R. M., 2004), in working memory (Khan & Muly, 2011), as well as in executive functions such as motor planning, inhibitory response control and sustained attention (Fibiger & Phillips, 1988); (Granon, et al., 2000); (Robbins, 2002).

More recently still, it was discovered that the heart secretes oxytocin, commonly referred to as the 'love' or bonding hormone. In addition to its functions in childbirth and lactation, recent evidence indicates that this hormone is also involved in cognition, tolerance, adaptation, complex sexual and maternal behaviours, learning social cues and the establishment of enduring pair bonds. Concentrations of oxytocin in the heart were found to be as high as those found in the brain (Gutkowska, Jankowski, Mukaddam-Daher, & McCann, 2000); (Cantin & Genest, 1986).

Furthermore, studies indicate that atrial peptide inhibits the release of stress hormones (Ströhle, Kellner, Holsboer, & Wiedemann, 1998), reduces sympathetic outflow (Butler, Senn, & Floras, 1994), plays a part in hormonal pathways that stimulate the function and growth of reproductive organs (Kentsch, Lawrenz, Ball, Gerzer, & Müller-Esch, 1992), and may even interact with the immune system (Vollmar, Lang, Hänze, & Schulz, 1990).

Even more intriguing, experiments suggest the atrial peptide can influence motivation and behaviour (Telegdy, 1994).

Heart-Felt Emotions – The Psychological Benefits

Beyond these findings, there is also a considerable body of other electrophysiological evidence demonstrating the modulation of higher brain activity by cardiovascular afferent input. Researchers have found that positive emotions such as appreciation and compassion, as opposed to negative emotions such as anxiety, anger, and fear, are reflected in a heart rhythm pattern that is more coherent. The coherent state has been correlated with a general sense of wellbeing, and improvements in cognitive, social and physical performance.

The Coherent Heart

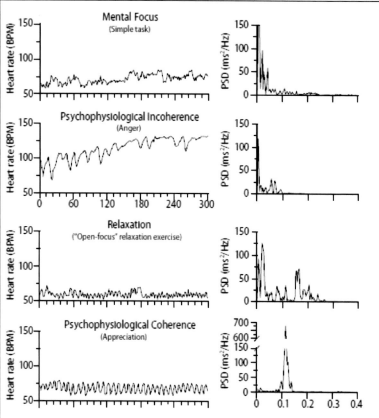

Emotions are reflected in heart rhythm patterns (as shown above).

The left-hand graphs are heart rate tachograms which show beat-to-beat changes in heart rate. To the right are the heart rate variability power spectral density (PSD) plots of the tachograms at left. The examples depicted are typical of the characteristic aspects of the more general patterns observed for each state.

Mental Focus is characterised by reduced HRV. Activity in all three frequency bands of the HRV power spectrum is present. Anger, an example of Psychophysiological Incoherence, characterised by a lower frequency, more disordered heart rhythm pattern and increasing mean heart rate. As can be seen in the corresponding power spectrum to the right, the rhythm during anger is primarily in the very low frequency region, which is associated with sympathetic nervous system activity.

Relaxation results in a higher frequency, lower amplitude rhythm, indicating reduced autonomic outflow. In this case, increased power in the high frequency region of the power spectrum is observed, reflecting increased parasympathetic activity (the relaxation response). Psychophysiological Coherence, which is associated with sustained positive emotions (in this example, appreciation), results in a highly ordered, sine-wave-like heart rhythm pattern. As can be seen in the corresponding power spectrum, this psychophysiological mode is associated with a large, narrow peak in the low frequency region, centered around 0.1 Hz.

Note the scale difference in the amplitude of the spectral peak during the coherence mode. This indicates system-wide resonance, increased synchronisation between the sympathetic and parasympathetic branches of the nervous system, and entrainment between the heart rhythm pattern, respiration, and blood pressure rhythms.

The coherence mode is also associated with increased parasympathetic activity, thus encompassing a key element of the relaxation response, yet it is physiologically distinct from relaxation because the system is oscillating at its resonant frequency, and there is increased harmony and synchronisation in nervous system and heart-brain dynamics.

(McCraty, Atkinson, Tomasino, & Bradley, 2006)

Data indicates that when heart rhythm patterns are coherent, the neural information sent to the brain facilitates cortical function. This effect is often experienced as heightened mental clarity, improved decision making and increased creativity. Additionally, coherent input from the heart tends to facilitate the experience of positive feeling states. This may explain why most people associate love and other positive feelings with the heart and why many people actually feel or sense these emotions in the area of the heart. So, the heart seems to be intimately involved in the generation of psychophysiological coherence (Tiller, McCraty, & Atkinson, 1996), (McCraty, 2000); (Lacey & Lacey, 1970); (McCraty, 2003b); and (Sandman, Walker, & Berka, 1982).

With every beat, the heart generates a powerful pressure wave that travels rapidly throughout the arteries, much faster than the actual flow of blood. These waves of pressure create what we feel as our pulse. The heart sounds, generated by the closing of the heart valves and cardiac murmurs, can be heard all over the chest and can extend as far as the groin.

Similarly, the pressure waves travelling through the arteries and tissues can affect every organ in the body, especially when the mechanisms that control blood pressure are compromised. In fact, the physical shock wave generated by the heartbeat expands the chest wall to such an extent that the heartbeat can be detected by measuring the chest expansion (this is called the ballistocardiogram). Important rhythms also exist in the oscillations of blood pressure waves.

In healthy individuals, a complex resonance occurs between blood pressure waves, respiration, and rhythms in the ANS. Because pressure wave patterns vary with the rhythmic activity of the heart, they represent yet another language though which the heart communicates with the rest of the body.

In essence, all of our cells sense the pressure waves generated by the heart and are dependent upon them in more than one way. At the most basic level, pressure waves force blood cells through the capillaries to provide oxygen and nutrients to the cells. In addition these waves expand the arteries, causing them to generate a relatively large electrical voltage. The waves also apply pressure to the cells in a rhythmic fashion, causing some of the proteins contained in them to generate an electrical current in response to the "squeeze."

All of these studies provide evidences to demonstrate the synchronisation of brain activity to the heart.

There is abundant evidence that emotions alter the activity of the body's physiological systems, and that beyond their pleasant subjective feeling, heart-felt positive emotions and attitudes provide a number of benefits that enhance physiological, psychological, and social functioning (Isen, 1998); (Fredrickson, 2002), (Wichers, et al., 2007).

As coherence tends to naturally emerge with the activation of heart-felt positive emotions such as appreciation, compassion, care and love, it suggests that such feelings increase the coherence and harmony in our energetic systems which are the primary drivers of our physiological systems (McCraty & Tamasino, 2006). This increased coherence and alignment in turn facilitate the body's natural regenerative processes.

"All nature is a continuum. The endless complexity of life is organized into patterns which repeat themselves – theme and variations – at each level of system. These similarities and differences are proper concerns for science."
(Miller, 1978)

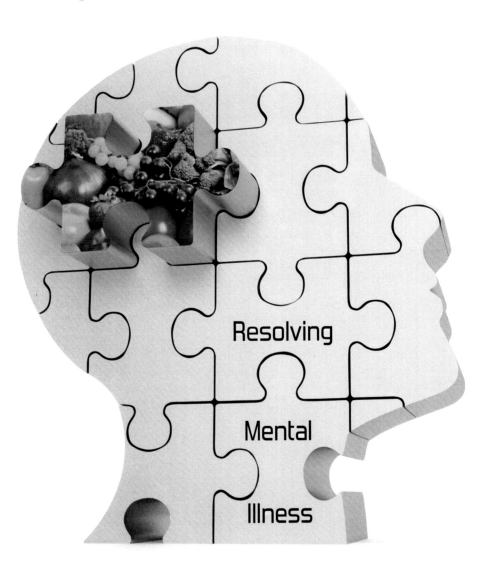

THERE ARE A number of treatment initiatives within the mental health sector, some of which I'll be mentioning in this section, but many of these initiatives are tokenistic at best.

Take, for example, an initiative due to be launched in 2014 encouraging international exchange between mental health experts. People are experts through experience, and this knowledge is accessible without having to go international – not that the project is of no benefit at all; there are people all over the world that have experienced mental illness. But I would strongly urge the decision-makers to think about what is going to make a <u>real</u> difference to the people that they claim they want to make a difference to. Nutritional therapy is nothing new but it is a crucial part of <u>real</u> recovery.

I'm not saying that nutritional therapy is the only option, nor am I saying that all other therapies and methods of treatment are of no benefit, but nutrition is an important part of everyone's wellbeing and, as has been shown, a significant part of recovery from illness – whether mental or physical.

Everyone eats, everyone can benefit, and particularly in the case of those that are already suffering mental health problems, it's about time they did.

Diverse Views on Recovery

As a survivor, I am aware that people from diverse backgrounds are or have been afflicted by mental disorders of varying degrees. Likewise, this diversity is also reflected in the diverse views on recovery. Although this is the case, most will agree on some key elements that signify or indicate that recovery is in progress or established.   Some service users have expressed their thoughts on recovery:

"It is about living well".

"It is about moving beyond diagnosis."

"It is about defining for yourself who you are rather than accepting how you have been defined by others."

Medication is only one of many tools for living well. Medication can be chosen for a short time (PRN), to deal with a crisis or for a longer time to prevent a crisis. Some people find it helpful, and some people do not. In recovery, the use of medication over the long term should be a matter of choice to facilitate the best long term mental health improvement and for successful (and consistent) recovery outcomes.

Millions of people with psychiatric diagnoses are living full and satisfying lives. But there is no 'one-size-fits-all' path called 'recovery'. What works for one person may not work for another. Recovery depends on unique needs and desired life and wellness outcomes.

People with a psychiatric diagnosis <u>can</u> get well and stay well, even from a 'major' illness like schizophrenia. Scientific studies demonstrate that a majority of individuals recover over time; while some individuals become free of psychiatric concerns altogether; others learn new ways of living and adjusting to the world.

It is also worth noting that some people have different definitions of recovery that may emphasise other factors, and these definitions may work better for them.

I HAVE WORKED within the mental health sector for many years, and I have learned important lessons from some of the patients for whom I've cared. I saw that some of them, instead of screaming and shouting, would find out about government legislation and mental health service policies for themselves; empowering <u>themselves</u> to take control of their treatment – shouting and screaming had gotten them nowhere and it would get me nowhere.

That's why I decided to conduct my own research into a cure, and, as you have seen, there is evidence out there. And not just out there; there's evidence within my own self and within other people that nutrition <u>does</u> make a difference – a big difference.

The body functions most optimally upon homeostasis, and it is constantly working to maintain this homeostasis – prioritising the vital organs, leeching nutrients from elsewhere when unavailable in the diet – so that sometimes imbalance can occur in the body as a result. Long-term use of pharmaceutical medication replicates the effect of poor diet – leeching nutrients from the rest of the body in order to function, eventually causing deficiency.

The answers are not always packaged in a bottle. Supplements can be helpful, no doubt, but if you can get nutrition from the food you eat, then that has all the properties – roughage, enzymes, etc. – that are needed to digest the food so that those nutrients can be absorbed and used efficiently.

The Importance of Homeostasis

Whenever any expert talks or writes about the human body's natural ability to heal itself, homeostasis is involved.

Maintaining balance in the body is essential to good health. And there is nothing more important to your physical health and mental wellbeing than eating well, sleeping well and drinking good water.

We all know that the conditions in the outside world change all the time. But things are different inside your body; the conditions in there hardly ever change at all.

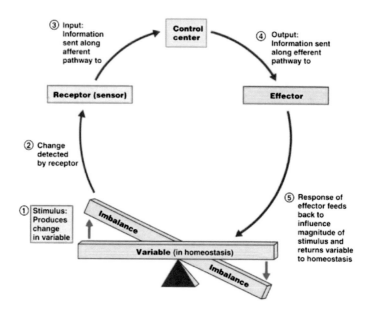

To maintain this 'sameness' which is called homeostasis, your body regulates itself in a number of ways. For example, the amount of carbon dioxide in the bloodstream is carefully controlled. The nervous system and hormones are responsible for this. Here are some of the other internal conditions that are controlled:

Blood sugar level

This is controlled to provide cells with a constant supply of energy. The blood sugar level is controlled by the release and storage of glucose, which is in turn controlled by a hormone called insulin.

Body temperature

This is controlled to maintain the temperature at which enzymes work best, which is 37°C. Body temperature is controlled by:

- controlling blood flow to the skin,
- sweating, and
- shivering.

The body's water content

This is controlled to protect cells by stopping too much water from entering or leaving them. Water content is controlled by water loss from:

- the lungs when we exhale,
- the skin by sweating, and
- the body, in urine produced by the kidneys

The human body is mainly water. This water is what assists in keeping the body in homeostasis so that the bodily processes function optimally, and the pH can be tested to measure how well a body is staying in equilibrium.

The pH, or potential hydrogen, is a scale between 0 and 14. If a body is functioning at its best, the pH will be close to 7, which is neutral. If a body is too acidic, it will be between 0 and 6.9, and if too alkaline, between 7.1 and 14.

The pH level may change temporarily after such activities as eating, but the actual pH will be evident over several periods of testing and getting close to the same results. Homeostasis affects the body's pH level, and therefore the health a person can maintain.

The human body is designed to heal itself. This cannot occur unless it is in a state of homeostasis, so the body will do what is necessary to try to maintain this balance. Calcium, potassium and sodium, which are alkalising minerals, will be taken from other areas of the body in order to keep this balance. Therefore, a person may end up with problems due to the decrease of these minerals, such as osteoporosis caused by the leeching of calcium from the bones.

Homeostasis and the Cells

All cells try to maintain constant internal conditions. One of the most critical elements of maintaining chemical balance within a cell is the cell membrane. All materials needed by the cell must move into the cell through the cell membrane; while all waste has to be discarded through it.

If materials such as water and minerals were to travel in and out of cells unregulated, cells would not maintain homeostasis. For this reason, cell membranes are selectively permeable. This means that only certain materials can cross the cell membrane.

There are two ways that materials can pass through the cell membrane:

One is called **diffusion/passive transport**, and requires no energy from the cell.

The other way is called **active transport** and requires energy from the cell.

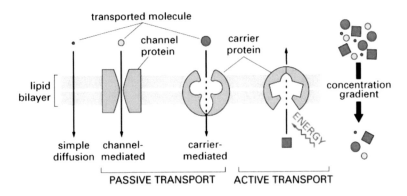

Diffusion/passive transport refers to the movement of material/molecules from an area of high concentration to an area of low concentration. This type of movement requires no energy; it is a spontaneous process.

Active transport refers to the movement of materials/molecules from an area of low concentration to an area of high concentration. This type of transport requires both a protein carrier and energy.

In both types of transport, materials squeeze through the tiny spaces between the molecules of the cell membrane.

The Roles Of Organ Systems In Homeostatic Regulation		
Internal Characteristics	Primary Organ Involved	Functions Of The Organ System
<u>Body temperature</u>	Integumentary system	Heat loss
	Muscular system	Heat protection
	Cardiovascular system	Heat distribution
	Nervous system	Coordination of blood flow, heat production, and heat loss

<u>Body fluid composition</u>		
Nutrient concentration	Digestive system	Nutrient absorption, storage, and release
	Cardiovascular system	Nutrient distribution
	Urinary system	Control of nutrient loss in the urine
Oxygen, carbon dioxide levels	Respiratory system	Absorption of oxygen, elimination of carbon dioxide
	Cardiovascular system	Internal transport of oxygen and carbon dioxide

Body fluid volume	Urinary system	Elimination or conservation of water from the blood
	Digestive system	Absorption of water, loss of water in faeces
	Integumentary system	Loss of water through perspiration
	Cardiovascular system	Distribution of water
Waste product concentration	Urinary system	Elimination of waste products from the blood
	Cardiovascular system	Transport of waste product to the sites of excretion

Blood pressure	Cardiovascular system	Pressure generated by the heart moves blood through blood vessels
	Nervous system and endocrine system	Adjustments in heart rate and blood vessel diameter can raise or lower blood pressure

Feedback Systems

Most feedback systems within the body are negative, meaning that change is bad news and needs to be countered.

Example of a basic feedback loop

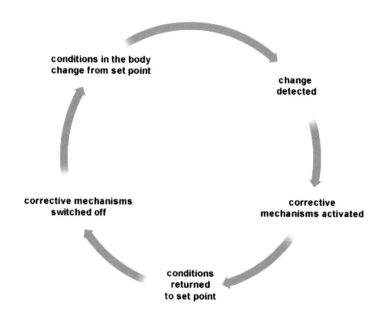

For example, in thermoregulation, it's the negative feedback that tells the hypothalamus when you're overheated and you need to sweat, or that you're really cold and need to shiver in order to generate heat.

Feedback can be positive too, meaning that the change in your body is a good thing, and should be increased for a while. One example of positive feedback is when a pregnant woman goes into labour. It's the positive feedback that controls the contractions to push the baby out.

Another part of the hypothalamus's job is to make you develop a fever when you're sick. At these times, your internal thermostat resets itself to a higher temperature which provides your body with more heat to fight infection.

Another example of homeostatic regulation is related to your excretory organs, which gets rid of chemical waste that could be poisonous to your body. Meanwhile, your immune system defends you from invading viruses, bacteria and allergens that don't belong in body.

There is also part of your brain called the respiratory centre, that makes sure you have the right oxygen and carbon dioxide mix in your blood at all times.

Short of trauma, stress is a huge factor which often interferes with homeostasis. Crucially, stress also frequently comes from eating the wrong foods. To counteract this, micronutrients from certain foods can help maintain the oxygen balance in your brain. They can help beneficial oxygen reach your brain as well as combat the highly-reactive forms of oxygen called free radicals.

All in all, homeostasis solves three basic internal environment problems:

1. excretion of metabolic wastes,
2. regulation of the concentration of ions and other chemicals, and

3. maintenance of water balance.

Homeostasis ensures that the environment inside your body remain stable regardless of the external changes. In this regard, homeostasis can be seen as part of the mind-body connection that regulates temperature, heart rate, blood pressure, and metabolism. These are only a few of nearly a thousand different internal variables which are automatically handled by the incredible mind-body alliance.

Importance of Maintaining Homeostasis

Homeostasis is a condition by which the biological/physical body is not lacking any nutrients and all needed nutritional components are readily available in their proper forms and amounts so every biological function can operate unimpeded.

The body needs to maintain homeostasis in order to stay alive; the internal environment of the body must stay relatively stable in order for the person to survive. It requires concentrations of nutrients, oxygen, and water to be normal and balanced, and for heat and pressure to be regulated at tolerable levels.

Both your brain and body function to their greatest potential when you make sure that your internal environment is healthy and stable. It is basic biology that your body maintains homeostasis when you give it the proper nutrition that it needs.

Critics seem particularly unable to consider that certain foods could produce mental illness. They think schizophrenia is confined to the brain. "How, then, could this important and isolated organ... be affected by the nutrition we feed our bodies? But, of course, the brain is entirely dependent on adequate, suitable nutrition (Bakker, 2010).

Excessive stress (in particular oxidative stress), poor diet, inadequate/excessive sleep, drugs, alcohol, smoking, poisons, or toxins create biochemical stress, leading to imbalances. These imbalances then negatively impact your cells' normal reactions and vital functions, creating mental and physical dysfunctions within the body. The remedy is to re-establish the balance.

Clearly, any therapeutic nutritional approach needs to be customised for each individual's condition(s), preferences and goals.

Nutritional Therapy – What's It All About?

Recent advances in research focusing on the influence of food on disease have shown how diet can be altered to impact symptoms and improve quality of life. Each one of us has different nutrient requirements depending on our current health, diet, lifestyle and our genes. Every cell in the body requires a precise balance of nutrients to function optimally, and that requirement changes as particular demands are made upon the body – as in the case of a chronic condition or hormonal change.

Nutritional therapy has proved particularly successful in alleviating certain chronic conditions and in reducing the risk of degenerative disease.

Nutritional therapy is the application of nutrition science in the promotion of health. It is recognised as a complementary medicine, and is relevant for individuals with chronic conditions as well as those looking for support to enhance their health and wellbeing.

The Case for Nutritional Therapy in Mental Health

Trace elements have been acting as intelligent ions for eons, long before scientists discovered their actions. They and other nutrients know exactly where to go in the body and what to do.

"For every drug that benefits a patient, there is a natural substance that can achieve the same effect."
(Pfeiffer's Law – Carl Pfeiffer Ph.D. MD.).

Drugs are different from nutrients; they are foreign to the body's natural biochemistry and thus produce side-effects. Nutrients are part of us, so side effects are minimal and seldom lethal.

With the nutritional approach to disease, the known blood or tissue levels and biochemical actions of each individual nutrient provide opportunities for objective measurement, the necessary yardstick for calculating the degree of impairment of the body, and the slow gradual improvement which occurs as the nutrients speed up normal biochemical processes. These objective signs are the keys to disease, from which we can learn exactly what is going on.

A balanced diet/nutrition and regular exercise can protect the brain and ward off mental disorders.

"Food is like a pharmaceutical compound that affects the brain."
(Fernando Gómez-Pinilla, UCLA professor of neurosurgery and physiological science)

"Diet, exercise and sleep have the potential to alter our brain health and mental function. This raises the exciting possibility that changes in diet are a viable strategy for enhancing cognitive abilities, protecting the brain from damage and counteracting the effects of ageing."
(Fernando Gómez-Pinilla)

Dr. Gómez-Pinilla analysed more than 160 studies about food's affect on the brain; the results of his analysis appear in the journal Nature Reviews Neuroscience (Wolpert, 2008).

Studies have shown that people suffering from schizophrenia and other mental disorders tend to consume diets that are lacking in essential nutrients.

Nutritional Therapies for Mental Disorders
(Lakhan & Vieira, 2008)

Abstract:

According to the Diagnostic and Statistical Manual of Mental Disorders, 4 out of the 10 leading causes of disability in the US and other developed countries are mental disorders.

Major depression, bipolar disorder, schizophrenia, and obsessive compulsive disorder (OCD) are among the most common mental disorders that currently plague numerous countries and have varying incidence rates from 26 percent in America to 4 percent in China.

Though some of this difference may be attributable to the manner in which individual healthcare providers diagnose mental disorders, this noticeable distribution can be also explained by studies which show that a lack of certain dietary nutrients contribute to the development of mental disorders. Notably, essential vitamins, minerals, and omega-3 fatty acids are often deficient in the general population in America and other developed countries; and are exceptionally deficient in patients suffering from mental disorders.

Studies have shown that daily supplements of vital nutrients often effectively reduce patients' symptoms. Supplements that contain amino acids also reduce symptoms, because they are converted to neurotransmitters that alleviate depression and other mental disorders.

Based on emerging scientific evidence, this form of nutritional supplement treatment may be appropriate for controlling major depression, bipolar disorder, schizophrenia and anxiety disorders, eating disorders, attention deficit disorder/attention deficit hyperactivity disorder (ADD/ADHD), addiction, and autism.

The aim of this manuscript is to emphasize which dietary supplements can aid the treatment of the four most common mental disorders currently affecting America and other developed countries: major depression, bipolar disorder, schizophrenia, and obsessive compulsive disorder (OCD).

Most antidepressants and other prescription drugs cause severe side effects, which usually discourage patients from taking their medications. Such noncompliant patients who have mental disorders are at a higher risk for committing suicide or being institutionalized. One way for psychiatrists to overcome this noncompliance is to educate themselves about alternative or complementary nutritional treatments.

Although, in the cases of certain nutrients, further research needs to be done to determine the best recommended doses of most nutritional supplements, psychiatrists can recommend doses of dietary supplements based on previous and current efficacious studies and then adjust the doses based on the results obtained.

"Orthomolecular psychiatry, a treatment strategy that uses megadoses of vitamins B_3 and C in conjunction with correct nutrition, yields a 90% recovery rate in acute cases and up to 50% in chronic patients."
(Hoffer, 1999).

Major Issues and Mounting Costs Of Mental Health

The W.H.O. predicts a 50% rise in child mental disorders by 2020.

Meanwhile, the UK Government has been forced to pump £342 million into school behaviour improvement programmes. Costs are mounting in the UK in relation to Mental Health as can be seen from government figures:

- In 2007 £77 billion
- In 2010 £105 billion

38% of Europeans ($\approx$165 million) have a fully developed mental or neorological illness (Wittchen, et al., 2011).

Most common mental health disorders	
Europe	Prevalence (Annual)
Anxiety Disorders	14.0%
Insomnia	7.0%
Major Depression	6.9%
Somatoform	6.3%
Alcohol and Drug dependence	5.4%
ADHD	5.0% in the young
Dementia	1-30% depending on age

"The time is now right for nutrition to become a mainstream, everyday component of mental health care."
(The Mental Health Foundation, 2006)

MY MESSAGE ISN'T about telling people to come off medication, that could produce symptoms even worse than the illness itself. My message is that people should be able to make that choice if that's what they want to do. To be able to do that they'd need to know what to replace medication with; to have something else to turn to, and to have support in that.

That support can take different forms. Families need to be educated so that they can know what to do – especially in the early, crucial stages. Often all a person needs is good quality rest, good quality nutrients, and to have people around them who are familiar. Being removed to a completely strange environment, away from family and friends, and forced to take medication that may have distressing side-effects is not always the answer. Putting someone without a mental illness into that scenario would undoubtedly cause significant distress, not to mention someone who is mentally unstable.

It's not a case of dismissing one therapy in favour of another; if we're going to talk about collaboration let's talk about <u>real</u> collaboration, with self-management and survivor-led services at the forefront. This nutritional, collaborative approach needs to be valued and taken seriously. When we talk about changes we need to talk about changes that are going to produce the outcomes service providers claim they want to achieve.

Recovery

Everyone has his/her own vision of "recovery" and that means having choices and the need to come together with peers; being treated as an expert about one's own life.

Recovery is about having a satisfying and fulfilling life, as defined by each person (Slade, 2009); (Repper & Perkins, 2003). Until relatively recently, it was assumed that most individuals with severe mental illness would never be "well" again (Kruger, 2000).

Recovery is probably the most important new direction for mental health services. It represents the convergence of a number of ideas such as:

- Empowerment
- Self-management
- Disability rights
- Social inclusion, and
- Rehabilitation

All this under a single heading that is supported by service users, mental health policy, authoritative sources and key leaders in mental health around the world.

Recovery ideas were given a strong impetus in the 1980s by evidence emerging from studies of the long-term outcomes of people with serious mental health conditions like schizophrenia. They challenged the idea that people would inevitably deteriorate, and demonstrated a wide range of different outcomes (Shepherd, Boardman, & Slade, 2008).

The 'recovery vision' or 'mental health recovery' (imported from the United States in 2002) is supposed to dramatically improve the lives of all individuals with mental illness, increasing independence, restoring hope and reducing social exclusion. It has been defined as a "highly individualized, strengths-based approach to symptom management" emphasizing "hope", "self-directed therapy, fitness, nutrition, peer support and spirituality." It also relies heavily on participation in programs such as the 'wellness recovery action plan' (WRAP) (The Wellesley Institute, 2009).

Support for Recovery

The recovery model is a social movement that is influencing mental health service development around the world. It refers to the subjective experience of optimism about outcome from psychosis, to a belief in the value of the empowerment of people with mental illness, and to a focus on services in which decisions about treatment are taken collaboratively with the user and which aim to find productive roles for people with mental illness. Flowing from this model is a renewed interest in educating service users about illness management (Warner, 2010).

Empowerment

"If any group of patients could benefit from being empowered by taking control of their own care, it is people with mental illness."
(Lamb, Press Release - More Choice in Mental Health, 2012)

"We will be asking the NHS to demonstrate real and meaningful progress towards achieving true 'parity of esteem' between mental health and physical care by March 2015."
(Lamb, NHS shakeup tackles disparity between mental and physical health services, 2012)

A central tenet of the recovery model is that empowerment of the user is important in achieving good outcome in serious mental illness. To understand why this may be so, it is important to appreciate that people with mental illness may feel disempowered, not only as a result of involuntary confinement or paternalistic treatment, but also by their own acceptance of the stereotype of a person with mental illness.

People who accept that they have a mental illness may feel driven to conform to an image of incapacity and worthlessness, becoming more socially withdrawn and adopting a disabled role. As a result, their symptoms may persist and they may become dependent on treatment providers and others. Thus, insight into one's illness may be rewarded with poor outcome.

This view is supported by an early study of people with serious mental illness which found that those who accept that they are mentally ill and have a sense of mastery over their lives (an internal locus of control) have the best outcomes. However, those who accept the label of mental illness tend to have lower self-esteem and an external locus of control, and those who find the mental illness label to be most stigmatising have the weakest sense of mastery.

Thus, internalised stigma undermines the possibility that insight will lead to a good outcome (Warner, 2010).

An important means of empowering patients is to involve them in decisions about their illness.

85% of clinicians believe that they share decisions about treatment with patients, but only 50% of patients believe this to be the case (Hibbard, Collins, & Baker, 2008).

"Empowerment of people with mental illness and helping them reduce their internalised sense of stigma are as important as helping them find insight into their illness. Until now, however, more effort has been expended on the last than on the former two factors."

(Warner, 2010)

Collaboration and Self-Management

Why collaborate?

"...there has been a failure to tackle the most important issue, namely the quality of interaction between patients and clinicians."
(Hibbard & Collins, 2008)

Collaboration is a process where two or more people work together towards a common goal with the purpose of improvement in health outcomes for the patient. Numerous randomised control trials give support to the view that the inclusion of the family and other carers in the patient's treatment results in improved outcomes for the patient, their carers and clinicians when using a collaborative approach.

The main outcomes include:

- A reduction in relapse rates (up to 20%) resulting in a reduced number of hospitalisations
- Better adherence to treatment
- Reduced psychiatric symptoms

Additional outcomes include:

- Improved social functioning of the service user
- Increased employment rates
- Increased involvement in the community
- Reduction in the burden experienced by family carers

- Improved relationship between family members, including improved relationship with the service user
- Cost effectiveness

Considerations for 'Collaborative Nutritional Therapy' to Become Part of Mental Health Service Delivery

Therapeutic interventions.

In managing people with complex mental health issues, no single therapy has been able to establish completeness of outcomes. Integrating evidence-based nutritional recommendations has a low risk to benefit ratio and will be an appealing proposal for those clinicians that recognise the need for integrated care.

What is integrated care?

Integrated care refers to a system where the patient's journey through the system of care is made as simple as possible.

"Care, which imposes the patient's perspective as the organising principle of service delivery and makes redundant old supply-driven models of care provision. Integrated care enables health and social care provision that is flexible, personalised, and seamless."
(Lloyd & Wait, 2006)

What is Collaborative Therapy and how does it work?

The Collaborative Therapy framework (Castle & Gilbert, 2006) looks at holistic treatment of people with mental illness. It has been widely acknowledged as a leading example of comprehensive service-user oriented care.

Collaborative Therapy is a comprehensive framework for service users, clinicians, services and others to work systematically towards the achievement of optimal mental health outcomes.

Collaborative Therapy as a Service Delivery Model provides:

- A series of workshops
- Manuals tested in practice, and
- Collaborative pathways to assist services in implementing the delivery model and evaluating the ongoing needs of service users and significant support networks.

The Collaborative Therapy framework has three components that can be applied across the spectrum of mental disorders. They encompass assessment/engagement, therapy sessions, and treatment integration using a service user-focused Collaborative Treatment Journal.

Assessment/Engagement

An integral part of Collaborative Therapy is the assessment/engagement component. The aim of the assessment is to screen for issues that may be barriers to treatment and to use this material to develop a pathway that will maximise the person's engagement in the service and Collaborative Therapy. The assessment also includes pre and post evaluation, such as service utilisation data to establish the effectiveness of Collaborative Therapy as a systems approach.

<u>The Therapy</u>

Structured intervention

The cornerstone of the therapy is one-on-one or group based work run over 8-12 weeks, followed by a relapse prevention component over a further 9 months. It is based on a newly designed version of the stress vulnerability model (Stress Vulnerability – Self Efficacy) and utilises consumer self-efficacy and self-reliance as part of the process.

The stress vulnerability model was proposed by Zubin and Spring (1977). It proposes that an individual has unique biological, psychological and social elements. These elements include strengths and vulnerabilities for dealing with stress. It provides core components of therapeutic interventions that have established efficacy across a wide range of diagnoses.

These consist of providing psychoeducation (psychoeducation is among the most effective of the evidence-based practices that have emerged in both clinical trials and community settings), coping and relapse prevention strategies, and other skills that can be usefully employed to manage mental health. Of particular importance, past research has highlighted self-efficacy and self-reliance as key components of improved mental health outcomes (Craig, Franklin, & Andrews, 1984); (Bandura, 1997).

Relapse prevention

The relapse prevention component is an integral part of the structured group or one-to-one therapy sessions and provides the basis for on-going adaptation and utilisation of skills learned in the initial intervention. This component involves the use of a specifically designed Collaborative Treatment Journal.

The Collaborative Treatment Journal (CTJ)

The CTJ is essentially a small pocket journal that can chart stressors, early warning signs, coping strategies, supports and other factors that influence the course and management of an individual's health. It is held by the service user and places the service user at the centre of their treatment by providing them with effective skills to maintain good health and the ability to facilitate good communication between themselves and others involved in the maintenance of their mental health (eg case managers, psychiatrists, GPs, Non-Government Organisation (NGOs) service providers).

In this way the journal knits together the various service sectors that service users engage with, and facilitates ongoing skills development, service user empowerment and service integration over time.

Self-Efficacy

Collaborative Therapy is based on self-efficacy. Self-efficacy essentially aims to place the person in control of their own illness and recovery by shifting the focus of the person's illness from being "dependent on" services to being "supported by" services. Self-efficacy is a systematic approach to both consumers and clinicians and underpins the whole framework of Collaborative Therapy. The CTJ is a fundamental component of the self-efficacy process.

Framework of Collaborative Therapy

The Collaborative Therapy framework allows ongoing identification of gaps and unmet needs in terms of service provision.

As a systems approach, it also has a built-in evaluation process at both an individual and service level, including risk management capabilities. It also provides a foundation for the development and evaluation of novel treatments, using robust scientific methodology. For example, data capture systems will allow for the identification of gaps and the development of interventions.

The unique appeal of the Collaborative Therapy framework is that it is sensitive to the structure, staff-mix and client-mix of individual services. This helps to ensure that there is maximum likelihood that the components developed within the Collaborative Therapy framework are adopted within routine service delivery (Berk, Berk, & Castle, 2004); (Bauer, et al., 1997); (Frogatt, Fadden, Johnson, Leggatt, & Shankar, 2007).

From Traditional To Collaborative Patient-Clinician Interactions

Traditional vs Collaborative Patient-Clinician Interactions
Adapted from Bodenheimer (2005)

Traditional Interactions		Collaborative Interactions
Information and skills are taught, based on the clinician's agenda	⟹	Patient and clinician share their agendas and collaboratively decide what information and skills are taught
There is belief that knowledge creates behaviour change	⟹	There is belief the one's own confidence in the ability to change ('self-efficacy'), together with knowledge, creates behaviour change

The patient believes it is the clinician's role to improve health	⟹ The patient believes that they have an active role to play in changing their own behaviours to improve their own health
Goals are set by the clinician and success is measured by compliance with them	⟹ The patient is supported by the clinician in defining their own goals. Success is measured by an ability to attain those goals.
Decisions are made by the clinician	⟹ Decisions are made as a patient-clinician partnership

Self-Management

There are a variety of definitions of self-management, and no universally accepted definition.

The term self-management is often misunderstood by patient, carer and psychiatrist. The terms 'self' and 'manage' suggest that the patient has ownership of their condition, and will be responsible for managing their condition in isolation and without assistance.

This is not the case. Self-management is the patient working in partnership with others, including health providers and carers to promote their health, manage their signs and symptoms, monitor behaviours and manage the impact of their condition. A good self-manager knows about their condition and is able to access resources and services to improve their every day quality of life.

An effective partnership or collaborative approach, where a psychiatrist works alongside the patient, carer and other health professionals to support the patient, ensures the best possible outcomes for the patient.

According to Improving Chronic Illness Care, self-management means: "...acknowledging the patients' central role in their care, one that fosters a sense of responsibility for their health. It includes the use of proven programs that provide basic information, emotional support, and strategies for living with chronic illness.

Self-management support can't begin and end with a class. Using a collaborative approach, providers and patients work together to define problems, set priorities, establish goals, create treatment plans and solve problems along the way," (Improving Chronic Illness Care, 2003).

"Self-management relates to the tasks that an individual must undertake to live well with one or more chronic conditions. These tasks include gaining confidence to deal with medical management, role management, and emotional management.

Self-management support is defined as the systematic provision of education and supportive interventions by health care staff to increase patients' skill and confidence in managing their health problems, including regular assessment of progress and problems, goal setting, and problem-solving support," (Adams, Greiner, & Corrigan, 2004).

In a qualitative study, Koch et al. (2004) outline three models of self-management:

1. The Medical Model that focuses on adherence
2. The Collaborative Model which proposes a partnership between individuals with chronic illness and health care professionals, and
3. The Self-agency Model that advocates self-determination.

The three models outline the continuum between traditional education and self-management education.

What is Self-management & Why is Self-Management Important?

Self-management is:

- Having knowledge of the illness and/or its management
- Adopting a self-management care plan agreed and negotiated in partnership with health

professionals, significant others and/or carers and supporters

- Actively sharing in decision-making with health professionals, significant others and/or carers and other supporters
- Monitoring and managing the signs and symptoms of the illness
- Managing the impact of the illness on physical, emotional, occupational and social functioning
- Adopting lifestyles that address risk factors and promote health by focusing on prevention and early intervention
- Having access to, and confidence in the ability to use support services.

According to Rethink Mental Illness: "An important part for many in the recovery journey is learning how to organise their life in a way which maximises good health and avoids triggers.

Successful self management will differ from person to person, as well as between mental illnesses, so it is important to remember that one size does not fit all. Many people find that learning as much as possible about their illness can be a great help," (Rethink Mental Illness).

"...providing treatment is not the primary purpose of mental health services. A recovery-oriented service supports people to use medication, other treatments and services as a resource in their own recovery."

(Slade, 2009)

According to David Crepaz-Keay, Head of Empowerment and Social Inclusion at the Mental Health Foundation: "Self-management is so important in empowering individuals to regain initiative, take control of their lives and put themselves back in the driving seat. An individual's mental health is a result of so many contributing factors and a holistic approach is vital in order to optimise and sustain recovery, (Mental Health Foundation, 2012)."

According to MIND: Self-management aims to increase your problem solving skills, boost your confidence and create more independence from psychiatric services. It's a set of skills learnt by groups of people to help manage struggles related to mental and physical wellbeing. This is done by setting and achieving your own goals (Lambeth and Southwark Mind).

Comparison of Traditional Education and Self-Management Education Adapted from Bodenheimer (2005)		
	Traditional Education	Self-Management ⟹ Education
<u>Content</u>	Disease specific and provides ⟹ information and technical skills related to the	Problem-solving skills to cope, manage and live with impact of living with a severe

	mental disorder	mental illness.
How the problem is defined	Inadequate control of the illness ⟹	Person with the mental illness formulates the problem, which may or may not be directly related to the illness.
Theoretical Constructs	Illness specific information leads to behaviour change, which then produces better clinical outcomes. ⟹	Greater self-efficacy, and increased confidence in the individual (learned through problem-solving skills and support) leads to improved clinical outcomes.
Goal	Compliance to prescribed behaviour change to improve clinical outcomes. ⟹	Increased self-efficacy for individuals improved clinical outcomes.
Educator	Health professional ⟹	Health professional, peer leader or people with lived experience of

	severe mental illness

Research Evidence Support for Self-Management

Support for self-management requires a focus on improving health and wellbeing and reducing health inequalities.

Here in the United Kingdom, the Expert Patients Programme is central to the chronic disease management policy. Like many other models now available, such as the Living a Healthy Life Course in New Zealand, the programme is an adaptation of the Chronic Disease Self-Management Program (CDSMP).

Early research work on the effectiveness of self-management was conducted at the Stanford Patient Education Research Centre, led by Professor Kate Lorig. Through extensive studies, Lorig and her team developed the CDSMP (Lorig, et al., 1999). The CDSMP has proven positive health outcomes for patients with genetic as well as illness-specific conditions. This includes reduced distress and increased self-efficacy.

A review of CDSMP studies by Gorden & Galloway (2008), found strong evidence to support a beneficial effect on physical and emotional outcomes and improvements in health-related quality of life.

Studies in a wide variety of chronic illnesses found that CDSMP patients show consistently greater energy/reduced fatigue, exercise more, have fewer social limitations, have increased psychological well-being, have enhanced partnerships with physicians, display improved health status and have greater self-efficacy.

In Australia, the Flinders Program of Self-Management is gaining significant recognition and has been endorsed by a number of Australian state departments of health and health service sectors as part of their efforts to reduce the burden of chronic disease.

The program includes a semi-structured assessment of self-management strengths and barriers and sets goals. A twelve-month care plan is created and agreed upon by the patient and the clinician, which incorporates medical and self-management actions.

Recent work by Lawn et al. (2007), using the patient-centred Flinders program, offers weight to self-management care planning being applicable to patients with mental illness. A feasibility study indicated that the Stanford CDSMP was applicable and acceptable to patients with serious mental illness as part of an overall self-management strategy, resulting in an improvement in self-management and mental functioning at three to six months follow-up.

Health care that is person/patient centred is focused on the needs, goals, beliefs and concerns of the individual rather than the needs of the system of health professionals. In this approach, the patient feels understood, appreciated and involved in the management of their condition.

Research supports the notion that people are empowered by learning skills and having the ability to gain control of their lives, and that this is preferable to others taking responsibility (Lawn & Battersby, 2009).

Common themes in patient-centred care have been identified as:

- Informing and involving patients
- Eliciting and respecting patient preferences
- Engaging patients in the care process
- Treating patients with dignity
- Designing care processes to suit patient needs – not providers
- Ready access to health information – both paper and electronic
- Continuity of care

The concept of 'expert patient' and 'shared decision-making' are models of patient-centred care. The Expert Patients Programme is an initiative implemented in the UK and the World Health Organization's 5 As framework (assess, advice, agree, assist and arrange) offers a systematic approach to shared decision-making.

There is growing evidence to support a patient-centred approach. Benefits have been determined as:

- Improved patient satisfaction
- Improved patient compliance and engagement in health process

- Reduced anxiety
- Improved quality of life
- Improved efficiency of care

A study by Swerrisen, in Victoria, Australia, has shown successful health outcomes when the CDSMP has been implemented with patients from Vietnamese, Chinese, Italian and Greek backgrounds. Participants in the intervention group had significantly better outcomes on energy, exercise, symptom management, self-efficacy, general health, pain, fatigue and health distress.

Similar change has been shown when the CDSMP has been delivered to patients in Shanghai and Hong Kong.

Overall, what these studies have shown is that many patients have a wealth of personal life experience of coping and recovering from chronic disease and severe mental illness, which can provide support for implementing self-management interventions.

The role of the care professional is to encourage self confidence and the capacity for self-management, and to support patients/service users to have more control of their conditions and their lives.

"Individuals often find the information and guidance needed to take more control over their care pathway lacking..."
(Peters, 2012)

"More work is needed to help people with serious mental illness such as bipolar disorder and schizophrenia to self-manage their disorder. Through self-management, many service users gain the confidence, skills and knowledge to better manage their mental health and gain more control of their lives at a time when they may feel they have lost control."

(Mental Health Foundation)

CONCLUDING THOUGHTS

Dr. Rachel Perkins OBE:

"The assumption that... professional 'experts' know best remains widespread (among both people using services and those providing them):

- professionals decide whether people need help ('gate-keeping' in services)

- professionals prescribe what is good for people and ensure their compliance – using the force of verbal persuasion and the force of the law if this fails.

Traditional services: one set of experts

- The expert professionals and the patients/clients/users: 'them' and 'us'

- Assumed that the expert professional has access to a body of knowledge that cannot be understood by non-experts

- Therefore it is the mental health workers' job to define people's reality – tell them what is wrong with them and what they should do... and get them to comply with/adhere to their prescriptions

Recovery-focused practice: two sets of experts

- Experts by profession, qualification and degrees – expertise based on professional research and theories

- Experts by lived experience – expertise based on personal experience and personal narratives

(Perkins, 2013)

This book reverberates voices such as those from the Schizophrenia Commission Report:

"...the system must give users and carers greater control and there must be accountability for individual outcomes. Professionals, policy makers and those who have experienced the system must work together in a spirit of respect and co-operation to bring about improvements."
(The Schizophrenia Comission, 2012)

The key message of this book is about embracing change and welcoming nutritional therapy as part and parcel of a genuine recovery treatment care-plan. It is my desire that this message serves to amplify, reflect, and validate the voices of many individuals (service users, carers, families and conscientious mental health professionals) calling for wider treatment choices and combinations, including naturally-derived treatments aimed at alleviating mental distress and suffering (particularly as it relates to the metabolic side-effects of new class medications).

Many sufferers (as well as their supporters) are not being made aware of the impact and value of essential nutrients as part of the recovery process. Due to this lack of vital information, as well as the absence of insights from a survivor perspective, many continue to experience unnecessary distress.

I also hope this book highlights the need for taking things to the next level; providing survivor-led (nutritional therapy-focused) recovery initiatives as part of meaningful changes towards working side by side with talk therapies.

He that takes medicine and neglects diet, wastes the skill of the physician.
(Chinese proverb)

The topics of nutritional issues and research findings herein add substantial weight and credence to the call for inclusion of nutritional therapy to bolster improvements in recovery and successful outcomes for mental disorders.

The findings presented in this book support and fall in line with current drives toward a collaborative approach, aimed at promoting self-directed recovery and self-management. As a survivor (someone with expertise by lived experience) I am acutely aware of the beneficial contribution that survivors like myself and others can bring to the table for progressing and taking forward the aims and objectives for genuine long-term recovery.

"People with psychosis also need to be given the hope that it is perfectly possible to live a fulfilling life after a diagnosis of schizophrenia or psychosis. We now need to make sure everyone is offered the treatments that we know work best... If we can achieve this, then together we can make the next decade one of increasing recovery..."

(Murray R. , 2012)

ACKNOWLEDGEMENTS

Abundant thanks to my wonderful daughter Camilah: without all of your hard work (checking and correcting my typo/spelling errors), your advice and support from start to finish; I don't know how I would have completed this book without you. I love you!

I also want to say a big thank you to my husband Abu Yusuf for being supportive and patient with the level of chaos and mess around the flat; with note papers and books scattered all around the living room.

I would also like to express my gratitude and love to my son Faruq and my daughter-in law Kameelah as well as my son-in-law Waseem for being there for me during very difficult periods of my illness (having concern for my health), and now trusting in my recovery. Also not forgetting my prodigal son Darren, who I pray will one day return.

Special expression of love to all of my grandchildren, and I pray that no one else in my family ever has to go through the horrors and distress of severe mental illness. This book is for you too!

Last, but not least, I would like to thank my colleagues at Rethink Mental Illness who have taken an interest and given me their support and encouragement by regularly asking me how the book is coming along and believing in my ability to write it.

I pray that this book has been of great benefit to everyone who has read it.

Thank you all.

APPENDICES

Appendix List

APPENDIX A
High Caffeine Use and Psychotic Symptoms – A Case Study

Caffeine, Mental Health, and Psychiatric Disorders

Caffeine intake is so common that its pharmacological effects on the mind are undervalued. Since it is so readily available, individuals can adjust their own dose, time of administration and dose intervals of caffeine, according to the perceived benefits and side effects of each dose.

Studies of caffeine in subjects with and without psychiatric disorders [show that], besides the possibility of mild drug dependence, caffeine may bring benefits that contribute to its widespread use. These benefits seem to be related to adaptation of mental energy to the context by increasing alertness, attention, and cognitive function (more evident in longer or more difficult tasks or situations of low arousal) and by elevating mood.

Accordingly, moderate caffeine intake (< 6 cups/day) has been associated with less depressive symptoms, fewer cognitive failures, and lower risk of suicide. However, its putative therapeutic effects on depression and ADHD have been insufficiently studied. Conversely, in rare cases high doses of caffeine can induce psychotic and manic symptoms, and more commonly, anxiety. Patients with panic disorder and performance social anxiety disorder seem to be particularly sensitive to the anxiogenic effects of caffeine, whereas preliminary data suggests that it may be effective for some patients with obsessive compulsive disorder (OCD).

(Lara, 2010)

Use of more than 300mg of caffeine daily might cause caffeine intoxication.

The symptoms include:

- Restlessness

- Nervousness

- Excitement

- Insomnia

- Flushed face

- Diuresis (increased urinary output)

- Gastrointestinal disurbance

- Muscle twitching

- Talking or thinking in a rambling manner

- Tachycardia (speeded-up heartbeat) or disturbances of heart rhythm

- Periods of inexhaustibility

- Psychomotor agitation

(Encyclopedia of Mental Disorders)

Most importantly, caffeine in combination with alcohol has heightened toxic effects, and this may be the culprit for deaths relating to caffeinated energy drinks. The caffeine is likely to offset the sedating effects of the alcohol and this allows for higher volumes of both substances to be ingested.

It is important to note what time of day caffeine is ingested so that effects on sleep can be minimised. The half-life for caffeine is 5 to 7 hours. This means that 5 to 7 hours after caffeine consumption, half of the caffeine has been metabolised by the liver and is eliminated from the body. For most people, one or two cups of coffee in the morning will not affect their sleep patterns later that evening.

People who consume caffeine regularly become dependent upon it and might experience lethargy and drowsiness without it. Since drinking coffee and caffeinated drinks is socially acceptable, use of it is a common occurrence. The individual who suddenly stops the use of these products is likely to have headaches for up to two weeks.

Caffeine is a stimulant that affects the central nervous system. It has mildly addictive properties and can lead to withdrawal symptoms for individuals who have daily caffeine uptake approximating 2 cups of coffee or more. Symptoms of withdrawal include:

- Anxiety

- Concentration difficulty

- Depressed mood

- Headache

- Irritability

Does Caffeine Interfere with Medications?

Caffeine can have adverse effects (by impairing absorption or increasing drug concentrations in the blood stream) when used in combination with the following medications and supplements:

Antibiotics

*Biaxin (clarithromycin), *Cipro (ciprofloxacin), *Erythromycin, *Norfloxacin, *Zithromax (azithromycin)

Psychiatric Medications

*Disulfiram, *Fluvoxamine, *Lithium, *Olanzapine

Other Medications

*Adenosine (cardiac), *Albuterol (asthma), *Cimetidine (antihistamine), *Echinacea (herbal), *Levothyroxine (thyroid), *Theophylline (asthma), *Vicodin (pain)

Overall, it is annoying to withdraw from caffeine but not dangerous. There is no reason to refrain from caffeine entirely unless you have specific risk factors as noted above. If you do choose to ingest caffeine, be sure to do so within safe limits, generally aiming for less than 300mg daily. You may need to decrease your caffeine intake if you are prescribed any of the medications noted above.

(Feke, 2013)

High Caffeine Use Linked to Psychotic Symptoms

ABC News Report, June 2011

A new study has found that high caffeine use, combined with stress, can cause people to exhibit psychotic symptoms such as hallucinations and delusions.

The research suggests that around five coffees, or the equivalent of 200mg of caffeine, may be enough to tip people over the edge and cause psychotic-like symptoms.

A team at Melbourne's La Trobe University were researching mechanisms between the onset of schizophrenia and stressful life situations.

They were trying to discover what caused stressed individuals who did not have a diagnosis of schizophrenia to show symptoms of the disease.

Lead researcher Simon Crowe says a sample of 92 undergraduate students were played White Christmas by Bing Crosby before being played static white noise for several minutes.

The students were then asked to press a buzzer to indicate when, if at all, they could hear White Christmas playing in the background of the white noise.

Lead researcher Simon Crowe says, however, White Christmas was never played during the white noise.

He says people who were both highly stressed and had a high intake of caffeine were three times more likely to report hearing the song.

"What we found was that people who are highly stressed and who are prone to high-level caffeine use are more likely to report these sorts of phenomena – hearing things that aren't necessarily there as a result of the interaction of those two effects," Professor Crowe said.

He says people who have a genetic predisposition to schizophrenia do not always show the disease, but it can be triggered by a number of things, including highly stressful situations.

"What caffeine does is increase the responsiveness of the system, which is made yet more powerful by [the presence of stress]," he said.

"It creates a situation where people tip further into the spectrum of 'highly stressed', and as a consequence they report these types of clinical phenomena."

Caffeine is the most commonly used psychoactive drug in the world and acts in the same way as other stimulant medications such as amphetamines.

Professor Crowe says as a result of our pressured lifestyles, Australia has become a stimulant-reliant society.

He says the situation needs to be looked at in greater detail.

"Caffeine is a drug that you can buy off the shelves, so it is an unregulated substance," he said.

"We are increasingly focused on how much things like alcohol and tobacco are available freely in the community, and here we have a stimulant – perhaps not as powerful as cocaine or amphetamine – which you can actually buy off the shelf at the supermarket."

(Grimson, 2011)

A Case Report of Caffeine-Induced psychosis

A 47-year-old successful male farmer with no history of psychiatric hospitalisation presented with a 7-year history of depression, diminished sleep to as little as 4 hours/night, poor energy, explosive anger, decreased concentration, decreased appetite, anhedonia, and feeling of worthlessness.

Seven years before his first presentation, the patient had developed the conviction that people were plotting against him to drive him off of his farm and take his land. At least twice, when he had found dead livestock on his farm, the patient thought that it was part of the plot against him and would entertain no other possibilities. The patient interpreted tyre tracks in the driveway as belonging to the car of individuals trying to take his land, even though other more plausible possibilities existed. According to the patient's wife, the subject interpreted many everyday occurrences as evidence of the plot.

Convinced of a plot against him, he installed surveillance cameras in his house and on his farm but never caught anything that would support his conviction that, as part of the plot, people were coming onto his farm at night. He became so preoccupied with the alleged plot that he neglected the business of the farm and eventually declared bankruptcy as a result. His preoccupation with the plot also led him to neglect the upkeep of his home, and he had his children taken from him because of unsanitary living conditions.

In addition to psychosis, the patient reported life-long difficulty sustaining attention, excessive talking, disorganisation, distraction, and forgetfulness. He denied other features of anxiety and psychosis. The patient reported drinking less than one case of beer annually. However, ~7 years before presentation, he had sharply increased his consumption of coffee from 10–12 cups/day to ~36 cups/day, a change in coffee consumption corroborated by his wife who made much of the coffee for him at home.

There was no history of psychosis before the increase in coffee consumption, but after the increased consumption, the patient developed paranoia. At presentation, the patient reported drinking >1 gallon of coffee/day.

At presentation, he was taking paroxetine 40 mg/day, alprazolam 0.5 mg TID, clonazepam 1 mg/day, and propranolol 10 mg QID. Medical history was remarkably only for hypertension. The mental status examination showed poor hygiene, but the patient was alert, oriented, friendly, and cooperative. Thought content showed paranoia. No medication changes were made, but the treating physician urged the patient to discontinue caffeine use.

At a 3-week follow-up, the patient said that he had reduced his caffeine intake by 50%. He was euthymic and much less paranoid. His hygiene was markedly improved. One month later, he had further reduced his coffee intake, had reduced his paroxetine to 20 mg/day, and was rarely using alprazolam. His mood continued to be euthymic and he was free from paranoia.

Two months later, he was drinking only 1–2 cups of coffee/day, paroxetine had been tapered and stopped, and he reported feeling better than he had for years. There was no evidence of paranoia or other psychosis. The surveillance cameras that he had installed earlier reportedly fell into disuse. Since the resolution of the original paranoia, the patient has at times increased his intake of caffeine, with a subsequent return of the paranoia, which has, in each case, resolved with reduced coffee intake.

DISCUSSION

While generally well tolerated, caffeine can be associated with a variety of adverse events, including depression. It is unknown whether the association between caffeine and depression is due to self-medication with caffeine to reduce depressive symptoms or a direct effect of caffeine from reduced mood. Moreover, caffeine in toxic doses can cause psychosis in otherwise psychiatrically healthy people and worsen psychosis in people with schizophrenia. Caffeine has been hypothesised to be a factor in some cases of clozapine-refractory psychosis.

In the case reported herein, the patient reported a ~7-year history of depression and psychosis that started after a sharp increase in caffeine use. He had no history of psychiatric hospitalisation to suggest a previous psychotic disorder and was using no other drugs associated with inducing psychosis, other than occasional alcohol use. While it is possible that the patient had an undiagnosed paranoid personality disorder, he had successfully operated his business, and his wife reported the onset of paranoia only after the increase of caffeine consumption.

Notably, with reduction of caffeine use and with no changes in his prescribed medications, the patient's mood improved and his paranoia was diminished at a follow-up visit 3 weeks later, making a paranoid personality disorder seem unlikely. Thereafter, he remained free of psychosis and depression.

After reducing his caffeine intake, the patient also began to decrease his alprazolam use. Considering the patient's report of a life-long history of problems sustaining attention, a tendency for distraction, disorganisation, and forgetfulness suggestive of attention-deficit/hyperactivity disorder, it may have been that the patient's use of caffeine, at least in part, was a self-medication attempt to improve attention and organisation. Regardless, in this case, we postulate that excessive consumption of caffeine may have been causally related to the development of psychosis, in that there is no evidence of psychosis antedating the heavy use of caffeine, and because the patient's psychosis resolved after he lowered his caffeine intake without the use of antipsychotic medication.

Adenosine inhibits serotonin and dopamine release; as such, by antagonising adenosine receptors, caffeine can increase dopaminergic effects. Accordingly, a reasonable explanation for the psychosis observed in this case is that the psychosis was due to elevated brain levels of dopamine from caffeine-induced adenosine antagonism. Because of caffeine's association with depression and anxiety, it is also possible that the patient's anxiety and depression were due to caffeinism as well.

CONCLUSION

In contrast to previous case reports that describe the acute occurrence of psychosis after heavy ingestion of caffeine, the case we report showed evidence of chronic psychosis that had resulted in severe psychosocial impairment and could easily have been mistaken for other long-term psychotic illness. Notably, the patient's psychosis resolved upon lowering caffeine intake, and no other features of schizophrenia or any other psychosis were present, sparing the patient from the potential adverse effects and cost of antipsychotic medication. Overall improvement in depression and anxiety also occurred when caffeine intake was lowered.

A single case report is not sufficient justification to recommend that chronic psychosis from caffeine consumption is common enough to be routinely inquired about in cases of chronic psychosis. However, based on the findings reported in this case, the relative ease of asking screening questions about caffeine use, and previous reports indicating that caffeine in high doses might cause psychosis, we suggest that caffeinism might be considered part of the differential diagnosis of chronic psychosis.

(Hedges, Woon, & Hoopes, 2009)

Dr. Hedges is an assistant professor in the Department of Psychology and the Neuroscience Center at Brigham Young University in Provo, Utah.

Mr. Woon is a doctoral student in clinical psychology in the Department of Psychology and the Neuroscience Center at Brigham Young University.

Dr. Hoopes is an adjunct faculty member in the Department of Psychiatry at the University of Utah School of Medicine and in private practice in Boise, Idaho.

Sources:

(Garrett & Griffiths, 1997)

(Fisone, Borgkvist, & Usiello, 2004)

(Nehlig, Daval, & Debry, 1992).

(Broderick & Benjamin, 2004)

(Nawrot, et al., 2003)

(Kruger, 1996)

(Dews, O'Brien, & Bergman, 2002)

(Wesensten, et al., 2002)

(Scott, et al., 2002)

(Yudofsky, Silver, & Hales, 1990)

(Diagnostic and Statistical Manual of Mental Disorders, 4th ed., 2000)

(Lucas, et al., 1990)

(Dratcu, Grandison, McKay, Bamidele, & Vasudevan, 2007)

(Paluska, 2003)

(Shaul, Farrell, & Maloney, 1984)

(Shen & D'Souza, 1979)

APPENDIX B
Evidence for Link between Psychological/Psychiatric Conditions and Omega-3

Abstract

AIM: Measure efficacy of eicosapentaenoic acid (EPA) in children with attention deficit hyperactivity disorder (ADHD).

METHODS: Randomized controlled trial (RCT) of 0.5g EPA or placebo (15weeks) in 92 children (7–12years) with ADHD. Efficacy measure was Conners' Parent/Teacher Rating Scales (CPRS/CTRS). Fatty acids were analysed in serum phospholipids and red blood cell membranes (RBC) at baseline and endpoint with gas chromatography.

RESULTS: EPA improved CTRS inattention/cognitive subscale (p=0.04), but not Conners' total score. In oppositional children (n=48), CTRS total score improved ≥25% in 48% of the children receiving EPA vs. 9% for placebo [effect size (ES) 0.63, p=0.01]. In less hyperactive/impulsive children (n=44), ≥25% improvement was seen in 36% vs. 18% (ES 0.41, n.s.), and with both these types of symptoms 8/13 with EPA vs. 1/9 for placebo improved ≥25% (p=0.03). Children responding to treatment had lower EPA concentrations (p=0.02), higher AA/EPA (p=0.005) and higher AA/DHA ratios (p=0.03) in serum at baseline. Similarly, AA/EPA (p=0.01), AA/DHA (p=0.038) and total Omega-6/omega-3 ratios (p=0.028) were higher in RBC, probably because of higher AA (p=0.011).

CONCLUSION: Two ADHD subgroups (oppositional and less hyperactive/impulsive children) improved after 15-week EPA treatment. Increasing EPA and decreasing Omega-6 fatty acid concentrations in phospholipids were related to clinical improvement.

(Gustafsson, et al., 2010)

Abstract

BACKGROUND: Developmental coordination disorder (DCD) affects ~5% of school-aged children. In addition to the core deficits in motor function, this condition is associated commonly with difficulties in learning, behaviour, and psychosocial adjustment that persist into adulthood. Mounting evidence suggests that a relative lack of certain polyunsaturated fatty acids may contribute to related neurodevelopmental and psychiatric disorders such as dyslexia and attention-deficit/hyperactivity disorder. Given the current lack of effective, evidence-based treatment options for DCD, the use of fatty acid supplements merits investigation.

METHODS: A randomized, controlled trial of dietary supplementation with omega-3 and omega-6 fatty acids, compared with placebo, was conducted with 117 children with DCD (5–12 years of age). Treatment for 3 months in parallel groups was followed by a 1-way crossover from placebo to active treatment for an additional 3 months.

RESULTS: No effect of treatment on motor skills was apparent, but significant improvements for active treatment versus placebo were found in reading, spelling, and behaviour over 3 months of treatment in parallel groups. After the crossover, similar changes were seen in the placebo-active group, whereas children continuing with active treatment maintained or improved their progress.

CONCLUSIONS: Fatty acid supplementation may offer a safe efficacious treatment option for educational and behavioural problems among children with DCD. Additional work is needed to investigate whether our inability to detect any improvement in motor skills reflects the measures used and to assess the durability of treatment effects on behaviour and academic progress.

(Richardson & Montgomery, 2005)

Abstract

Schizophrenia is associated with a broad range of neurodevelopmental, structural and behavioural abnormalities that often progress with or without treatment. Evidence indicates that such neurodevelopmental abnormalities may result from defective genes and/or non-genetic factors such as pre-natal and neonatal infections, birth complications, famines, maternal malnutrition, drug and alcohol abuse, season of birth, sex, birth order and life style. Experimentally, these factors have been found to cause the cellular metabolic stress that often results in oxidative stress, such as increased cellular levels of reactive oxygen species (ROS) over the antioxidant capacity. This can trigger the oxidative cell damage (i.e., DNA breaks, protein inactivation, altered gene expression, loss of membrane lipid-bound essential polyunsaturated fatty acids [EPUFAs] and often apoptosis) contributing to abnormal neural growth and differentiation. The brain is preferentially susceptible to oxidative damage since it is under very high oxygen tension and highly enriched in ROS susceptible proteins, lipids and poor DNA repair. Evidence is increasing for increased oxidative stress and cell damage in Schizophrenia. Furthermore, treatments with some anti-psychotics together with the lifestyle and dietary patterns, that are pro-oxidant, can exacerbate the oxidative cell damage and trigger progression of neuropathology. Therefore, adjunctive use of dietary antioxidants and EPUFAs, which are known to regulate the growth factors and neuroplasticity, can effectively improve the clinical outcome. The dietary supplementation of either antioxidants or EPUFAs, particularly omega-3 has already been found to improve some psychopathologies. However, a combination of antioxidants and omega-3 EPUFAs, particularly in the early stages of illness, when brain has high degree of neuroplasticity, potentially may be even more effective for long-term improved clinical outcome of Schizophrenia.

(Mahadik, Pillai, Joshi, & Foster, 2006)

Abstract

OBJECTIVES: Research has linked eating disturbances with behavioural impulsivity. Little is known, however, about whether eating disturbances and aggressive behaviour have a tendency to co-occur in the same girls. This article assesses the eating disturbance-aggressive behaviour association and then examines the extent to which these factors confer a risk on drug use and attempted suicide.

METHOD: Survey data were gathered from 3,630 girls in grades 6 through 12 in the upper Midwest. Girls responded anonymously to questions regarding binge eating and purging, dietary restriction, aggressive behaviour, drug use, and attempted suicide. Logistic regression analysis was used to assess the unique contribution of demographic variables, eating disturbances, and aggression on drug use and attempted suicide.

RESULTS: Eating disturbances were significantly associated with aggressive behaviour. Girls who endorsed binge eating and purging or dietary restriction had odds of aggressive behaviour 2 to 4 times higher than girls who did not endorse these items. Logistic regression revealed that eating disturbances and aggressive behaviour were significantly associated with both drug use and attempted suicide.

CONCLUSIONS: Eating disturbances are significantly associated with aggressive conduct in adolescent girls. The constellation of eating disturbances and aggressive behaviour is associated with a greater risk of drug use and attempted suicide.

(Thompson, Wonderlich, Crosby, & Mitchell, 1999)

Abstract

BACKGROUND: There is evidence that offenders consume diets lacking in essential nutrients and this could adversely affect their behaviour.

AIMS: To test empirically if physiologically adequate intakes of vitamins, minerals and essential fatty acids cause a reduction in antisocial behaviour.

METHOD: Experimental, double-blind, placebo-controlled, randomised trial of nutritional supplements on 231 young adult prisoners, comparing disciplinary offences before and during supplementation.

RESULTS: Compared with placebos, those receiving the active capsules committed an average of 26.3% (95% CI 8.3-44.33%) fewer offences (P=0.03, two-tailed). Compared to baseline, the effect on those taking active supplements for a minimum of 2 weeks (n=172) was an average 35.1% (95% CI 16.3-53.9%) reduction of offences (P<0.001, two-tailed), whereas placebos remained within standard error.

CONCLUSIONS: Antisocial behaviour in prisons, including violence, are reduced by vitamins, minerals and essential fatty acids with similar implications for those eating poor diets in the community.

(Gesch, Hammond, Hampson, Eves, & Crowder, 2002)

APPENDIX C
Schizophrenia and Nutritional Studies

Schizophrenia is a mental disorder that disrupts a person's normal perception of reality. Schizophrenic patients usually suffer from hallucinations, paranoia, delusions, and speech/thinking impairments. These symptoms are typically presented during adolescence.

Dietary Factors – Low Saturated Fat Observational study

The statistical association between the average ratings of the course and outcome of schizophrenia in 8 national centres (participating in the World Health Organization international 2-year follow-up study) and the amount of fat in the average national diet was investigated. In order to study the influence of the types of fat consumed, fats were subdivided into those composed predominately of saturated fat (derived from land animals and birds) and fat having a relatively high content of unsaturated fatty acids (derived from vegetables, fish, and seafood).

A high intake of total fat as well as of saturated fat was significantly associated with unfavourable ratings of the course and outcome of schizophrenia. The intake of unsaturated fat was not significantly correlated with any of the ratings, although a trend suggested that a high intake of unsaturated fat may be associated with favourable ratings.

97% of the variation in the overall outcome of schizophrenia between the national centres could be explained by the combined variation in the percentages of fat from land animals and birds and from vegetables, fish, and seafood, respectively, in the national diets.

(Christensen & Christensen, 1988)

Remove Caffeine – Review Article

There are 3 reports of psychotic episodes being precipitated by excessive caffeine use, and reports which describe psychotic episodes following treatment with pharmacologic agents containing large amounts of caffeine. Usually, the patient begins to experience anxiety and then begins to markedly increase caffeine consumption, resulting in greater anxiety or psychosis. In addition, a study of caffeine use on a psychiatric ward indicated that high users of caffeine tended to have more psychotic symptomatology.

Caffeine is a methylxanthine that is absorbed approximately 1 hour after ingestion and has a serum half-life of 3 hours. Animal studies suggest that it can both release norepinephrine and increase norepinephrine synthesis in the CNS. It also appears to increase brain serotonin and has a biphasic effect on dopamine, with an initial increase followed by a prolonged decrease.

(Mikkelsen, 1978); (McManamy & Schube, 1936)

Vitamins-Folic Acid 2mg. Daily

May be deficient. Observation study 17/47 patients (36%) with schizophrenia (DSM III) referred as out-patients, or as candidates for psychiatric hospitalisation had borderline (red-cell folate < 200 micrograms/l) or definite (red-cell folate <150 micrograms/l) folate deficiency.

(Godfrey, et al., 1990)

May be reduced in "histapenic" as compared to "pyroluric" schizophrenics.

Observational Study: The average serum folate in 10 "histapenic" schizophrenics (patients with low histamine and high copper levels) was 6.0 ±3.1 ng/ml compared to 12.3 ±6.2 ng/ml in 26 "pyroluric" schizophrenics (normal in copper but deficient in pyridoxine and zinc).

(Pfeiffer & Braverman, 1979).

Experimental study: In a retrospective survey, 13/36 patients with schizophrenia or endogenous depression and low serum folate levels had been treated with folic acid in addition to standard treatment. Treated and untreated patients did not differ significantly on age and sex distributions. 12/13 (92.3%) folate-treated patients made a full social recovery (either with or without residual symptoms) vs. 16/23 (69.6%) controls. Of 13 patients with schizophrenia who were hospitalised 10 or more days, the folate-treated patients averaged 44.3 days while the 10 controls averaged 70.1 days, a significant difference.

(Carney, 1979); (Reynolds, 1975)

Experimental Study: Folic acid, along with vitamin B_{12}, niacin, vitamin C and zinc, was effective in the treatment of "histapenic" schizophrenics resulting in reduction in serum copper and rise in blood histamine after 5-6 months along with symptomatic improvement. On the other hand, folic acid worsened patients with high histamine and normal copper levels ("histadelic" schizophrenics) who responded to mild antifolate drugs, such as phenytoin, and agents that decrease histamine, such as calcium salts and methionine, in doses of 1-2 gm/day.

(Pfeiffer & Braverman, 1979).

Supplementation with folic acid may be beneficial.

Warning: Supplementation with folic acid can cause an exacerbation of psychotic behaviour if blood levels become elevated.

Thiamine

Supplementation may be beneficial by activating pyruvate dehydrogenase in the brain. With acetazolamide – a drug which inhibits carbonic anhydrase, the enzyme which catalyzes the hydration of carbon dioxide and dehydration of carbonic acid. Combined administration may be beneficial.

Experimental Double-Blind Study: 24 patients with chronic schizophrenia disorders for at least 4 years, who had failed to improve with traditional therapy, were given acetazolamide daily and thiamine 500mg 3 times daily with meals or placebo. After 8 weeks, only patients in the experimental group showed significant improvement including a 17% improvement in hallucinations, 14% in delusions, 25% in bizarre behaviour, and 16% in positive formal thought disorder. 50% of patients in the experimental group showed improvement on both of the two assessment scales. No neurological side effects were noted.

(Sacks, Esser, Feitel, & Abbott, 1989).

<u>Vitamin C</u>

Reduced dietary intake may be associated with the risk of schizophrenia.

Observational study: In a comparison of the population of 3 areas in Croatia which differed in schizophrenia prevalence rate, the population with the highest schizophrenia rate had a significantly lower ascorbic acid intake, and 60% of the examined families had an unsatisfactory vitamin C consumption compared to 10% of families in the population with the lowest schizophrenia rate.

(Suboticanec, 1986).

Plasma levels may be depressed, even with intakes considered to be adequate for normals.

Observational study: Compared to hospitalised neurotics, hospitalised schizophrenics were found to have a lower average vitamin C plasma level.

(Suboticanec, 1986).

Observational study: 20 hospitalised schizophrenics and 15 controls received the same diet containing an average of 50mg ascorbic acid daily. After at least 2 months, the average plasma vitamin C level in the schizophrenics was significantly lower (p<0.05).

(Suboticanec, 1986).

Observational study: The average plasma vitamin C level in 885 hospitalised psychiatric patients was 0.51/100ml compared to 0.87/100ml in 110 healthy controls. 32% of the patients had levels below 0.35 mg/100 ml, the threshold which has been associated with detrimental effects on immune responses and behaviour.

(Schorah, Morgan, & Hullin, 1983).

<u>Fatty Acids</u>

Supplementation may be beneficial: 5 patients were treated with linseed oil (50% alpha-linolenic acid) which was individually titrated in the range of 2-6 tbsp daily (0.2-1.0 g/kg/d) in divided doses depending upon response. The 2 patients with a history of remissions and relapses responded; only 1 of the 3 patients with no-relapsing illness appeared to gain any benefit. The responding patients also had other signs and symptoms (drying dermatoses, automatic neuropathies, tinnitus, fatigue) which suggested that they were suffering from a deficiency of omega-3 fatty acids which provide the substrate upon which niacin and other B vitamin holoenzymes act to form the prostaglandin 3 series hormones.

(Rudin, 1981).

Review article: Schizophrenia is associated with clinical phenomena that can be explained by disturbances in polyunsaturated fatty acid and prostaglandin metabolism. Since decreased PGE_1 (a prostaglandin) activity can be associated with increased dopamine release, PGE_1 deficiency is consistent with the dopamine hypothesis of schizophrenia.

(van Kammen, Yao, & Goetz, 1989)

Supplementation may be beneficial.

Experimental Double-Blind Study: 38 hospitalised patients, primarily schizophrenics, who had been exposed to neuroleptics for a long period of time and had established movement disorders were treated either with evening primrose oil (Efamol) 12 caps daily (each containing 45mg GLA and 360mg linoleic acid) or with placebo. After 16 weeks, there were highly significant improvements to total psychopathology scores and schizophrenia subscale scores, and a significant improvement in memory. The antidyskinetic effect was marginally significant but not clinically important.

(Vaddadi, Courtney, Gilleard, Manku, & Horrobin, 1989).

Nutrition And Schizophrenia: Beyond Omega-3 Fatty Acids

(Peet, 2004)

Abstract

There are now five placebo-controlled trials of EPA in the treatment in schizophrenia, and four of these have given positive or partly positive findings. A cross-national ecological analysis of international variations in outcome of schizophrenia in relation to national dietary practices, showed that high consumption of sugar and of saturated fat is associated with a worse long-term outcome of schizophrenia. It is known that a high sugar, high fat diet leads to reduced brain expression of brain-derived neurotrophic factor (BDNF) which is responsible for maintaining the outgrowth of dendrites.

Low brain BDNF levels also lead to insulin resistance which

occurs in schizophrenia and is associated with diseases of the metabolic syndrome. It appears that the same dietary factors which are associated with the metabolic syndrome, including high saturated fat, high glycaemic load, and low omega-3 PUFA, may also be detrimental to the symptoms of schizophrenia, possibly through a common mechanism involving BDNF.

Amino Acids

Disturbances in amino acid metabolism have been implicated in the pathophysiology of schizophrenia. Specifically, an impaired synthesis of serotonin in the central nervous system has been found in schizophrenic patients.

(van der Heijden, et al., 2005).

Other Studies

High doses (30 g) of glycine have been shown to reduce the more subtle symptoms of schizophrenia, such as social withdrawal, emotional flatness, and apathy, which do not respond to most of the existing medications.

(Javitt, Zylberman, Zukin, Heresco-Levy, & Lindenmayer, 1994)

(Leiderman, Zylberman, Zukin, Cooper, & Javitt, 1996); (Javitt, et al., 2001).

An open-label clinical trial performed in 1996 revealed that 60 g of glycine per day (0.8 g/kg) could be given to schizophrenic patients without producing adverse side effects and that this dose led to a two-fold increase in cerebrospinal fluid (CSF) glycine levels.

(Leiderman, Zylberman, Zukin, Cooper, & Javitt, 1996).

A second clinical study treated patients with the same dosage divided into 3 doses within 1 week. This form of glycine treatment led to an eight-fold increase in CSF glycine levels.

(Javitt, et al., 2001)

The most consistent correlation found in one study that involved the ecological analysis of schizophrenia and diet, concluded that increased consumption of refined sugar results in an overall decreased state of mind for schizophrenic patients, as measured by both the number of days spent in the hospital and poor social functioning.

(Peet, 2004b)

That study also concluded that the dietary predictors of the outcome of schizophrenia and prevalence of depression are similar to those that predict illnesses such as coronary heart disease and diabetes.

A Danish study showed that better prognoses for schizophrenic patients strongly correlate with living in a country where there is a high consumption of omega-3 fatty acids.

(Christensen & Christensen, 1988).

Eicosapentaenoic acid (EPA), which is found in omega-3 fish oils, has been shown to help depressive patients and can also be used to treat schizophrenia.

(Peet, 2003)

Furthermore, studies suggest that supplements such as:

- 280 milligrams of EPA from marine omega-3 fish oil
- 100 milligrams of organic virgin evening primrose omega-6 oil
- 1 milligram of the anti-oxidant vitamin E

when taken on a daily basis, helps healthy individuals and schizophrenic patients maintain a balanced mood and improves blood circulation. For schizophrenic patients, docosahexaenoic acid (DHA) supplements inhibit the effects of EPA supplements so it is recommended that the patient only takes the EPA supplement, which the body will convert into the amount DHA it needs.

(Peet, 2003)

(Emsley, Myburgh, Oosthuizen, & van Rensburg, 2002)

(Puri, et al., 2000)

(Richardson, Easton, Gruzelier, & Puri, 1999)

(Richardson, Easton, & Puri, 2000)

(Richardson, 2003)

(Yao, et al., 2004)

Double-blind, placebo controlled studies, randomized, placebo controlled studies, and open-label clinical studies have all shown that approximately 2 g of EPA taken daily in addition to one's existing medication effectively decreases symptoms in schizophrenic patients.

(Peet, 2003)

(Emsley, Myburgh, Oosthuizen, & van Rensburg, 2002)

(Yao, et al., 2004)

APPENDIX D
An Interview: Dr Bonnet Discusses Pyroluria

An Interview with Dr. Phillip Bonnet on the Subject of Pyroluria.

(The Healing Partnership)

Interviewer: Dr. Bonnet, can you define pyroluria for us?

Dr. Bonnet: Pyroluria is a metabolic disorder in which, under conditions of stress, a person becomes functionally depleted of pyridoxine (vitamin B6) and zinc. It was first identified in the late 1950's through tests with psychiatric patients in a psychiatric hospital. Through a specific laboratory test of the patient's urine, what has become known as the mauve-factor was identified.

In 1963 Doctors Abram Hoffer and Humphrey Osmond coined the name 'malvaria' for those patients who had a mauve factor in their urine. Extensive testing showed that the mauve factor occurred in about one out of three confined in a psychiatric hospital.

Interviewer: When and how did you become involved in this research?

Dr. Bonnet: I joined the research team of Dr. Osmond and Dr. Carl C. Pfeiffer at the New Jersey Neuro-Psychiatric Institute in 1972. By that time Dr. Pfeiffer had seen some astounding results of his experimental research. Particularly in a young lady, named Sara. Sara had come to the Institute in terrible shape. She was fifteen years old at the time, and was suffering from seizures, chronic insomnia and had bouts of amnesia and vomiting. She was at the point where she clearly wanted to die. The laboratory tests showed her urine to have a strong mauve factor and high coproporphyrin excretion. Her psychiatric rating test (the EWI [Experiential World Inventory]) clearly showed considerable perceptive disorder. Sara was given large doses of vitamin B6 (up to 1 gm per day), along with supplementary zinc (160mg) and 8 mg of manganese; she responded immediately. In fact, Sara's recovery was so dramatic, she applied to and was accepted not only to college but went on to a successful modelling career. Today she continues a maintenance dosage of the vitamin and mineral supplements to prevent a relapse, but leads a healthy, sane life. Dr. Pfeiffer originally called the condition the "Sara Syndrome." Today it is referred to by the more generic term pyroluria.

My continued study, research and interest in the topic, stems from my personal diagnosis of pyroluria. I have maintained a dosage of about 1500mg. of B6 for years. Only recently, when I expanded my practice to include homeopathic remedies, have I experienced such a remarkable improvement that I now maintain a dosage of 250mg of B_6.

Interviewer: You noted that initially psychiatric patients were identified as having pyroluria. Is the problem limited to psychiatric patients?

Dr. Bonnet: No. In trying to identify its origin we found pyroluria definitely showed genetic roots. In fact, although the disorder can be inherited from only one parent, most of the time both parents have the disorder. In fact there is a better than 50/50 chance of this happening. It is also seen in geniuses. In fact, both Emily Dickinson and Charles Darwin had all of the classic symptoms of pyroluria.

Interviewer: You raise an important point. What are the symptoms?

Dr. Bonnet: The diagnosis of pyroluria is fairly easy to make. Symptoms include:

1. Poor stress tolerance. This is often first noticed as a student completes high school and leaves homes for the more competitive world of college or a career. Stress levels skyrocket beyond previous (safe within the confines of the family) levels. With college students, symptoms are usually seen to be cyclical in that they increase and decrease with the cycle of the workload within the semester. Most crises usually surface as the end of the semester approaches.
2. A tendency to not be hungry for breakfast, sometimes even experiencing morning nausea.
3. Infrequent recall of dreams upon awakening. This does not mean necessarily being able to relay the dreams, but to remember dreaming.
4. Pain in the left upper quadrant of the body. This is because the spleen is congested. B_6 is necessary to stabilise the red blood cell membranes, and when a person is deficient in B_6, the red cells turn over more rapidly than normal and that leads to congestion of spleen.
5. History of mild anaemia that doesn't respond to iron.
6. A tendency for skin to burn easily in the sun.

Examining the patient is likely to reveal: white spots on the fingernails; paleness (of complexion); and crowded incisors.

A word of caution: although the symptoms seem fairly easy to identify by the patient, it can be dangerous to self-diagnose and self-treat. Incorrect large doses of B_6 can be dangerous and a proper balance of zinc (generally gluconate) is required.

Interviewer: How would the diagnosis be confirmed?

Dr. Bonnet: Final determination of the disorder requires a urine test. This determines the Urinary Ehrlich Chromphor (UEC) level.

Considerable care must be taken in gathering the urine. Due to the fact that the substance we are looking for is very unstable and quite vulnerable to decomposing, my office adds ascorbic acid to specimen as soon as the patient voids. The specimen is then frozen over dry ice. This is critical and must be enforced for a correct reading. Our lab is likewise extremely careful of temperature when administering the test.

Interviewer: Once the diagnosis has been determined, what is the procedure for treating the disorder? Will the patient be able to return to or continue a "normal" life?

Dr. Bonnet: Following usual treatment protocol, the patient starts with a dosage of 500mg. of the B_6. We adjust it upwards by 250mg. every four days until the person starts to recall dreaming on a regular basis. If they dream too much on the 500mg, we cut back on that dosage. Sometimes if a person is dreaming too much on even 250mg it could be an indication that they don't have pyroluria.

Usually pyroluric people require doses between 250 to 1500mg. Some require up to 2000mg. And there is an occasional patient that does need more. In the past we always had to keep a close watch on the dosage, especially watching for a more serious side effect – numbness in the toes, called peripheral neuropathy – with pyridoxine (the standard form of B6). However by adding Pyridoxal-5-Phosphate (P-5-P), the active form of vi,tamin B6 we have been able to prevent the peripheral neuropathy and maintain a much lower amount of vitamin B_6. The neuropathy comes about because of an imbalance between pyridoxine and P-5-P; taking additional P-5-P takes care of the problem. Hence, it has been a long time since we have seen people with numb toes.

Interviewer: Are there any other symptoms that a patient should report regarding pyroluria?

Dr. Bonnet: Some pyroluric patients will find they cannot handle any level of outside involvement with people. The stress of these situations is unbearable. In severe cases, the stress reaches the point that the patient spends their time in seclusion. The patient might also report blinding headaches, nervous exhaustion, a change in handwriting and familial dependency. Both Charles Darwin and Emily Dickinson were known to have these symptoms. Dramatic personality as well as physical changes are generally seen when the disorder is properly treated. The patient will return to a healthy happy life, often finding a job if they are not working, or being promoted if they are employed. When pyroluria is very severe, there can be an abnormal (unpleasant sweetish) odour to the person's breath. In a psychiatric patient, this usually indicates a breakdown is pending. The reason for this odour is not currently known, but continuing research is being conducted.

Frequently gastrointestinal problems are also noted – particularly irritable bowel syndrome and colitis (that can be anything from spastic colon to ulcerative colitis). Episodes of diarrhoea and constipation also indicate a lack of B_6. Some seizure disorders can be traced to pyroluria.

One more note, B_6 is known as the asthma nutrient. People with pyroluria will sometimes come down with asthmatic difficulties. We have also seen increased instances of arthritic disorders as well.

Interviewer: Pyroluria, although first identified in psychiatric patients, certainly does not seem to be limited to that population. You have made it clear why this problem needs to be diagnosed at your office, where careful patient history and proper testing of the urine can be handled. Are there any other guidelines for patients to follow?

Dr. Bonnet: The most important guideline for any patient to follow is adequate nutrition and practicing a lifestyle of moderation in all activities (both work and play). Learn to LOVE your body and take care of it with the proper respect.

Natural treatments for depression involve the identification of nutritional imbalances, allergies and yeast overgrowth. Supplements like St. John's Wort, SAMe and essential fatty acids have proven to be very helpful, while the use of medications is sometimes necessary.

APPENDIX E
Bacteria & the Brain: The Powerful Behaviour-Modifying Effects of the Gut

(McEvoy, 2013)

The gut has been called "the second brain". Research reveals that the enteric nervous system (ENS), a branch of the autonomic nervous system that is found in the GI tract, can communicate with, and function independently of the brain. The enteric nervous system of the gut is comprised of about 500 million neurons. The enteric nervous system can "think", "remember" and "learn" on its own accord.

The enteric nervous system lines the mucosa of various organs: oesophagus, stomach, small intestine, large intestine, pancreas, gall bladder, and biliary tree.

The ENS is involved in the regulation of several essential digestive functions. Most notably:

- Peristalsis, intestinal motility: bowel muscular contractions

- Digestive enzyme secretion: to break down food particles

- Participates in the regulation of oesophageal muscles: moving food to your stomach

- Motility of the gall bladder, releasing bile into the duodenum

- Assists the hormone secreting in releasing pancreatic enzymes

- Exchange of fluids and electrolytes in the gut

- Blood flow through the gastric mucosa

- Also involved in the regulation of the gastric and oesophageal sphincters: preventing acid food from entering the throat, and allowing food to pass into the duodenum from the stomach

- Uses more than 30 neurotransmitters, including serotonin, GABA, dopamine, acetylcholine

Many researchers postulate that the enteric neurons have an important role to play in regulating behaviour. This is likely due to the fact that the enteric nervous system communicates with the brain via the vagus nerve. It is known that strains of intestinal bacteria have a powerful regulatory effect on the enteric neurons. It is also known that these same bacterial colonies can induce behaviour-modifying effects.

In 2011, researchers from the Journal of Neurogastroenterology stated: *"As Bifidobacterium longum decreases excitability of enteric neurons, it may signal to the central nervous system by activating vagal pathways at the level of the enteric nervous system."*

What this means is that behaviour is directly linked to intestinal bacteria and gut function.

Behaviour & Leaky Gut

It is now well established that gut permeability, known as "leaky gut" has a direct effect on behaviour. Studies such as this have demonstrated the link between intestinal permeability, gut infections and depression.

A key mechanism with how intestinal permeability plays a crucial role in behavioural disorders is mostly due to the effect that pathogens and bacterial species have on brain and neurotransmitter function.   For example, streptococcal infections have been shown to cause symptoms of OCD (obsessive compulsive disorder), tics, and Tourette's. Additionally, the immune response that is invoked from strep and other infections, causes tremendous systemic inflammation including to that of the brain.

The outer casing of gram-negative bacteria, known as lipo-polysaccharides (LPS), has shown in studies to induce massive systemic inflammation, including the release of pro-inflammatory cytokines such as TNF-a in the brain, as well as brain microglial activation.

Because of the essential role of "tight junctions" in the gut lining for protecting the organism from invading antigens, a diminishment of the tight junctions leads to an increased level of permeability, allowing various pathogenic microbes easy access into circulation. This permeability of the gut wall induces high levels of inflammatory activity in the brain, nervous system and in many other locations in the body.

Additionally, leaky gut will also feature imbalanced gut flora, especially in the presence of pathogens and with an overgrowth of opportunistic organisms. This may involve imbalances in the same gut bacteria that communicate with the brain via the vagus nerve. So, behaviour and brain function are affected by the gut in more than one way.

The Role of Intestinal Flora in Modifying Behaviour: Gut Microbiome Axis

The intestinal flora makes up roughly 80% of the total immune defences of the body. The gut is lined with more than 100 trillion micro-organisms, nearly ten times the amount of cells that make up the human body. There are thought to be between 400-1000 different species of bacteria that are normally found in the gut, and there exist intrinsic relationships and complex communication networks among the bacterial species.

Immediately following birth, the act of breastfeeding results in the implantation of essential floral colonies into the infant's gut. Studies have demonstrated that breast feeding significantly reduces the risk of childhood asthma. Breast feeding for more than 12 months has been shown to be protective against the development of rheumatoid arthritis. One study found a correlation between a shorter duration of breast feeding and the development of ADHD in children.

Many recent studies have focused on the role that certain probiotic strains have on regulating behaviour. This is fascinating because it shows the relationship between bacteria and the brain. The probiotic strain bifido infantis 35624 has been studied for its role in possibly reducing depression. Additionally, bifido infantis powerfully reduces IBS (Irritable Bowel Syndrome) symptoms.

Lactobacillus reuteri has been studied for its anti-anxiety effects and for its powerful modulation of the immune system, especially the inhibition of TNF-a. Additionally, L-reuteri is well established to modify the activity of the neurotransmitter GABA in the CNS. The same is true for lactobacillus rhamnosus.

L-helveticus and B-longum have been studied for effectively reducing stress, anxiety and depression.

There are a plethora of additional studies that demonstrate the role of gut microbes in regulating behaviour.

Without a doubt, continual research will emerge that identifies the intricate but profound role that bacterial balance in the gut plays at modifying behaviour.

Repair the Gut: Reduce Inflammation, Improve Cognition

Any serious health-improvement program should address the function of the gut flora and mucosal barrier. This is magnified exponentially if one has chronic gut issues, inflammatory conditions, autoimmune disorders, and behavioural issues.

Because there are so many factors that will impede upon your intestinal flora, maintaining proper digestion, assimilation and intestinal immunity is paramount. All of these factors work together.

It is extremely common that when the gut is severely compromised, the mucosal barrier is damaged, and the "tight junctions" that normally exist to keep pathogens at bay are compromised. If this is the case, there will most likely be a greater degree of inflammation that can manifest at places in the body you wouldn't necessarily suspect (such as the brain).

Often accompanying gut flora imbalances are food intolerances of varying degrees. In fact, food allergies and sensitivities may be amplified when one's gut flora is compromised. For some individuals eliminating gluten, dairy and eggs may be essential. For others, low-oxalate diets may be important.

In many instances, it may take years of persistent attention to the gut before long-term results are achieved.

It is the opinion of this author, from firsthand experience, that proper, individualised nutrition is the foundation for restoring the function of the gut mucosal barrier.

Michael McEvoy has a private nutritional consulting practice. He works with clients nationally and internationally. Please contact him to learn more about his nutritional consulting services and programs.

APPENDIX F
Suicide Attempts Linked to Inflammatory Chemical

(Pappas, 2012)

A chemical in the brain may explain why some people become suicidal — and it may link inflammation of the body to disorders of the mind.

According to new research, suicidal individuals have elevated levels of quinolinic acid in the fluid surrounding the CNS. "The discovery could explain a missing link between inflammation and mental illness", said study researcher Lena Brundin, a professor of translational science and molecular medicine at Michigan State University. Previously, scientists had linked suicidal feelings to the kind of bodily inflammation that occurs during illness or stress, but they weren't able to explain how inflammation could translate to depression, hopelessness and a desire to kill oneself.

The new study of 100 Swedish patients finds that the higher the level of quinolinic acid in the spinal fluid, the stronger their desire to commit suicide.

Brundin said: "The sicker the patient, the higher the quinolinic acid."

WORKS CITED

Adams, K., Greiner, A. C., & Corrigan, J. M. (2004). *The 1st Annual Crossing the Quality Chasm Summit: A Focus on Communities.* Washington DC: National Academies Press.

Aleman, A., Hijman, R., de Haan, E. H., & Kahn, R. S. (1999). Memory impairment in schizophrenia: A meta-analysis. *The American Journal of Psychiatry, 156*(9), 1358-1366.

Alhola, P., & Polo-Kantola, P. (2007). Sleep deprivation: Impact on cognitive performance. *Neuropsychiatric Disease and Treatment, 3*(5), 553-567.

American Psychiatric Association. (2000). *Diagnostic and Statistical Manual of Mental Disorders, 4th ed.* Washington DC: American Psychiatric Association.

Appleton, K. M., Hayward, R. C., Gunnell, D., Peters, T. J., Rogers, P. J., Kessler, D., & Ness, A. R. (2006). Effects of n-3 long-chain polyunsaturated fatty acids on depressed mood: Systematic review of published trials. *The American Journal of Clinical Nutrition, 84*(6), 1308-1316.

Armour, J. A. (1991). Anatomy and function of the intrathoracic neurons regulating the mammalian heart. In I. H. Zucker, & J. P. Gilmore, *Reflex Control of the Circulation* (pp. 1-37). Boca Raton: CRC Press.

Armour, J. A. (1994). *Neurocardiology: Anatomical and Functional Principles.* New York: Oxford University Press.

Armour, J. A. (2004). Cardiac neuronal hierarchy in health and disease. *American Journal of Physiology. Regulatory, Integrative and Comparative Physiology, 287*(2), R262-271.

Armour, J. A., & Kember, G. C. (2004). Cardiac sensory neurons. In J. A. Armour, & J. L. Ardell, *Basic and Clinical Neurocardiology* (pp. 49-117). New York: Oxford University Press.

Arvindakshan, M., Ghate, M., Ranjekar, P. K., Evans, D. R., & Mahadik, S. P. (2003). Supplementation with a combination of omega-3 fatty acids and antioxidants (vitamins E and C) improves the outcome of schizophrenia. *Schizophrenia Research, 62*(3), 195-204.

Auslander, L. A., & Jeste, D. V. (2002). Perceptions of problems and needs for service among middle-aged and elderly outpatients with schizophrenia and related psychotic disorders. *Community Mental Health Journal, 38*(5), 391-402.

Bakker, E. (2010). *Violence and Nutrition.* Retrieved from Naturopath: http://www.naturopath.co.nz/Nutrition/Violence+and+Nutrition.html

Bandura, A. (1997). The anatomy of stages of change. *American Journal of Health Promotion, 12*(1), 8-10.

Bauer, M. S., McBride, L., Shea, N., Gavin, C., Holden, F., & Kendall, S. (1997). Impact of an easy-access VA clinic-based program for patients with bipolar disorder. *Psychiatric Services, 48*(4), 491-496.

Becker, E. S. (2010). Obesity and mental illness in a representative sample of young women. In P. Killeen, *Addiction: The Hidden Epidemic.* Xlibris Corporation.

Beitman, B. D., & Dunner, D. L. (1982). L-tryptophan in the maintenance treatment of bipolar II manic-depressive illness. *The American Journal of Psychiatry, 139*(11), 1498-1499.

Benton, D. (1990). The impact of increasing blood glucose on psychological functioning. *Biological Psychology, 30,* 13-19.

Berk, M., Berk, L., & Castle, D. (2004). A collaborative approach to the treatment alliance in bipolar disorder. *Bipolar Disorders, 6*(6), 504-518.

Bhatia, H. S., Agrawal, R., Sharma, S., Huo, Y. X., Ying, Z., & Gomez-Pinilla, F. (2011). Omega-3 fatty acid deficiency during brain maturation reduces neuronal and behavioural plasticity in adulthood. *PLoS One*, e28451.

Blackburn, G. L. (2000). Weight gain and antipsychotic medication. *The Journal of Clinical Psychiatry, 61*(Suppl. 8), 36-41.

Bodenheimer, T., MacGregor, K., & Sharifi, C. (2005, June). *Helping Patients Manage Their Chronic Conditions.* Retrieved from California Healtcare Foundation: http://www.chcf.org/~/media/MEDIA%20LIBRARY%20Files/PDF/H/PDF%20HelpingPatientsManageTheirChronicConditions.pdf

Bohm, D., & Hiley, B. J. (1993). *The Undivided Universe.* London: Routledge.

Bowden, C. L., Huang, L. G., Javors, M. A., Johnson, J. M., Seleshi, E., McIntyre, K., . . . Maas, J. W. (1988). Calcium function in affective disorders and healthy controls. *Biological Psychiatry, 23*(4), 367-376.

Brenna, J. T., Salem, N. J., Sinclair, A. J., & Cunnane, S. C. (2009). *Official Policy Statement Number 5: a-Linolenic Acid Supplementation and Conversion to n-3 Long Chain Polyunsaturated Fatty Acids in Humans.* ISSFAL.

Brewerton, T. D., & Reus, V. I. (1983). Lithium carbonate and L-tryptophan in the treatment of bipolar and schizoaffective disorders. *The American Journal of Psychiatry, 140*(6), 757-760.

Broderick, P., & Benjamin, A. B. (2004). Caffeine and psychiatric symptoms: A review. *The Journal of the Oklahoma State Medical Association, 97*(12), 538-542.

Bromundt, V., Köster, M., Georgiev-Kill, A., Opwis, K., Wirz-Justice, A., Stoppe, G., & Cajochen, C. (2011). Sleep-wake cycles and cognitive functioning in schizophrenia. *The British Journal of Psychiatry, 198*(4), 269-276.

Brown, A. S. (2008). The risk for schizophrenia from childhood and adult infections. *The American Journal of Psychiatry, 165*(1), 7-10.

Brown, A. S., Begg, M. D., Gravenstein, S., Schaefer, C. A., Wyatt, R. J., Bresnahan, M., . . . Susser, E. S. (2004). Serologic evidence of prenatal influenza in the etiology of schizophrenia. *Archives of General Psychiatry, 61*(8), 774-780.

Brown, S. (1997). Excess mortality of schizophrenia. A meta-analysis. *The British Journal of Psychiatry, 171*, 502-508.

Buka, S. L., Goldstein, J. M., Seidman, L. J., & Tsuang, M. T. (2000). Maternal recall of pregnancy history: Accuracy and bias in schizophrenia research. *Schizophrenia Bulletin, 26*(2), 335-350.

Butler, G. C., Senn, B. L., & Floras, J. S. (1994). Influence of atrial natriuretic factor on heart rate variability in normal men. *The American Journal of Physiology, 267*(2 Pt 2), H500-505.

Cagampang, F. R., & Bruce, K. D. (2012). The role of the circadian clock system in nutrition and metabolism. *The British Journal of Nutrition, 108*(3), 381-392.

Campbell-McBride, N. (2004). *Gut and Psychology Syndrome.* Cambridge: Medinform Publishing.

Cantin, M., & Genest, J. (1986). The heart as an endocrine gland. *Scientific American, 254*(2), 76-81.

Carman, J. S., & Wyatt, R. J. (1979). Calcium: Bivalent cation in the bivalent psychoses. *Biological Psychiatry, 14*(2), 295-336.

Carney, M. W. (1979). Psychiatric aspects of folate deficiency. In M. I. Botez, & E. N. Reynolds, *Folic Acid in Neurology, Psychiatry and Internal Medicine.* New York: Raven Press.

Castle, D. J., & Gilbert, M. (2006). Collaborative therapy: Framework for mental health. *The British Journal of Psychiatry, 189,* 467.

Chee, M. W., & Chuah, L. Y. (2008). Functional neuroimaging insights into how sleep and sleep deprivation affect memory and cognition. *Current Opinion in Neurology, 21*(4), 417-423.

Chernigovskiy, V. N. (1967). *Interceptors: Russian Monographs on Brain and Behavior, 4.* Washington DC: American Psychological Association.

Chouinard, G., Beauclair, L., Geiser, R., & Etienne, P. (1990). A pilot study of magnesium aspartate hydrochloride

(Magnesiocard) as a mood stabilizer for rapid cycling bipolar affective disorder patients. *Progress in Neuropsychopharmacology & Biological Psychiatry, 14*(2), 171-180.

Chouinard, G., Young, S. N., & Annable, L. (1985). A controlled clinical trial of L-tryptophan in acute mania. *Biological Psychiatry, 20*(5), 546-557.

Christensen, O., & Christensen, E. (1988). Fat consumption and schizophrenia. *Acta Psychiatrica Scandinavica, 78*(5), 587-591.

Cohrs, S. (2008). Sleep disturbances in patients with schizophrenia: Impact and effect of antipsychotics. *CNS Drugs, 22*(11), 939-962.

Colantuoni, C., Rada, P., Patten, C., Avena, N. M., Chadeayne, A., & Hoebel, B. G. (2002). Evidence that intermittent, excessive sugar intake causes endogenous opioid dependence. *Obesity Research, 10*(6), 478-488.

Coleridge, H. M., Coleridge, J. C., & Rosenthal, F. (1976). Prolonged inactivation of cortical pyramidal tract neurones in cats by distension of the carotid sinus. *The Journal of Physiology, 256*(3), 635-649.

Costa, E., Dong, E., Grayson, D. R., Guidotti, A., Ruzicka, W., & Veldic, M. (2007). Reviewing the role of DNA (cytosine-5) methyltransferase overexpression in the cortical GABAergic dysfunction associated with psychosis vulnerability. *Epigenetics, 2*(1), 29-36.

Craig, A. R., Franklin, J. A., & Andrews, G. (1984). A scale to measure locus of control of behaviour. *The British Journal of Medical Psychology, 57*(Pt 2), 173-180.

Cunnane, S., Drevon, C., Spector, A., Sinclair, A., & Harris, B. (2004). *ISSFAL Board Statement Number 3: Recommendations for intake of polyunsaturated fatty acids in healthy adults.* Brighton: ISSFAL.

Dalman, C., Allebeck, P., Gunnell, D., Harrison, G., Kristensson, K., Lewis, G., . . . Karlsson, H. (2008). Infections in the CNS during childhood and the risk of subsequent psychotic illness: A cohort study of more than one million Swedish subjects. *The American Journal of Psychiatry, 165*(1), 59-65.

Davies, S., & Stewart, A. (1987). *Nutritional Medicine.* London: Pan Books.

Demar, J. C., Ma, K., Bell, J. M., Igarashi, M., Greenstein, D., & Rapoport, S. I. (2006). One generation of n-3 polyunsaturated fatty acid deprivation increases depression and aggression test scores in rats. *Journal of Lipid Research, 47*(1), 172-180.

Dews, P. B., O'Brien, C. P., & Bergman, J. (2002). Caffeine: Behavioral effects of withdrawal and related issues. *Food and Chemical Toxicology, 40*(9), 1257-1261.

Downey, M. (2012, June). *Life Extenstion Magazine Report: New Reason to Avoid Stress.* Retrieved from Life Extension:

http://www.lef.org/magazine/mag2012/jun2012_New-
Reason-Avoid-Stress_01.htm

Dr. Andrews, W. H. (2011, August 12). Telomeres and Ageing.
Retrieved from
http://www.youtube.com/watch?v=x1zw6uRxKYU

Dr. Berk, M. (2011, September 15). *Inflammatory Cause of
Bipolar Disorder Suggests New Treatments.* (M. L.
Zoler, Ed.) Retrieved from Clinical Psychiatry News:
http://www.clinicalpsychiatrynews.com/news/more-
top-news/single-view/inflammatory-cause-of-bipolar-
disorder-suggests-new-treatments/fac7f33968.html

Dr. Cohen, S. (2012, April 2). *Press Release: How Stress
Influences Disease: Carnegie Mellon Study Reveals
Inflammation as the Culprit.* Retrieved from Carnegie
Mellon University:
http://www.cmu.edu/news/stories/archives/2012/april
/april2_stressdisease.html

Dr. Lustig, R. (2011, March 24). Sugar: The Bitter Truth.
Retrieved from
http://www.youtube.com/watch?v=0z5X0i92OZQ

Dratcu, L., Grandison, A., McKay, G., Bamidele, A., &
Vasudevan, V. (2007). Clozapine-resistant psychosis,
smoking, and caffeine: managing the neglected
effects of substances that our patients consume every
day. *American Journal of Therapeutics, 14*(3), 314-318.

Drinkhill, M. J., & Mary, D. A. (1989). The effect of
stimulation of the atrial receptors on plasma cortisol

level in the dog. *The Journal of Physiology, 413*, 299-313.

Dubovsky, S. L., Christiano, J., Daniell, L. C., Franks, R. D., Murphy, J., Adler, L., . . . Harris, R. A. (1989). Increased platelet intracellular calcium concentration in patients with bipolar affective disorders. *Archives of General Psychiatry, 46*(7), 632-638.

Edwin, E., Holten, K., Norum, K. R., Schrumpf, A., & Skaug, O. E. (1965). Vitamin B12 hypovitaminosis in mental diseases. *Acta Medica Scandinavica, 177*, 689-699.

Emsley, R., Myburgh, C., Oosthuizen, P., & van Rensburg, S. J. (2002). Randomized, placebo-controlled study of ethyl-eicosapentaenoic acid as supplemental treatment in schizophrenia. *The American Journal of Psychiatry, 159*(9), 1596-1598.

Encyclopedia of Mental Disorders. (n.d.). *Caffeine-related disorders.* Retrieved June 2013, from Encyclopedia of Mental Disorders: http://www.minddisorders.com/Br-Del/Caffeine-related-disorders.html

Epel, E. S. (2009). Psychological and metabolic stress: A recipe for accelerated cellular ageing? *Hormones (Athens, Greece), 8*(1), 7-22.

Esterling, B. A., Kiecolt-Glaser, J. K., Bodnar, J. C., & Glaser, R. (1994). Chronic stress, social support, and persistent alterations in the natural killer cell response to cytokines in older adults. *Health Psychology, 13*(4), 291-298.

Fairclough, S. H., & Houston, K. (2004). A metabolic measure of mental effort. *Biological Psychology, 66,* 177-190.

Farmer, P. (2012, December 13). *Press Release - More Choice in Mental Health.* Retrieved from GOV.UK: https://www.gov.uk/government/news/more-choice-in-mental-health

Feke, T. (2013, January 7). *Caffeine Pros and Cons.* Retrieved from Dr. Tanya Feke: http://www.tanyafeke.com/?p=2235

Fellerhoff, B., Laumbacher, B., Mueller, N., Gu, S., & Wank, R. (2007). Associations between Chlamydophila infections, schizophrenia and risk of HLA-A10. *Molecular Psychiatry, 12*(3), 264-272.

Fibiger, H. C., & Phillips, A. G. (1988). Mesocorticolimbic dopamine systems and reward. *Annals of the New York Academy of Sciences, 537,* 206-215.

Fisone, G., Borgkvist, A., & Usiello, A. (2004). Caffeine as a psychomotor stimulant: Mechanism of action. *Cellular and Molecular Life Sciences, 61*(7-8), 857-872.

Forest, G., Poulin, J., Daoust, A. M., lussier, I., Stip, E., & Godbout, R. (2007). Attention and non-REM sleep in neuroleptic-naive persons with schizophrenia and control participants. *Psychiatry Research, 149*(1-3), 33-40.

Forster, A., & Stone, T. W. (1976). Evidence for a cardiovascular modulation of central neuronal activity in man. *Experimental Neurology, 51*(1), 141-149.

Fredrickson, B. L. (2002). Positive emotions. In C. R. Snyder, & S. J. Lopez, *Handbook of Positive Psychology* (pp. 120-134). New York: Oxford University Press.

Freeman, M. P., Hibbeln, J. R., Wisner, K. L., Davis, J. M., Mischoulon, D., Peet, M., . . . Stoll, A. L. (2006). Omega-3 fatty acids: evidence basis for treatment and future research in psychiatry. *The Journal of Clinical Psychiatry, 67*(12), 1954-1967.

Frogatt, D., Fadden, G., Johnson, D. L., Leggatt, M., & Shankar, R. (2007). *Families as Partners in Mental Health Care: A Guidebook for Implementing Family Work.* Toronto: World Fellowship for Schizophrenia and Allied Disorders.

Fuller, P. M., Lu, J., & Saper, C. B. (2008). Differential rescue of light-and food-entrainable cirdadian rhythms. *Science, 320*(5879), 1074-1077.

Ganguli, R. (2012, June 26-28). Antipsychotics and weight gain. *Hot Topics Conference on Obesity and Mental Health.*

Garrett, B. E., & Griffiths, R. R. (1997). The role of dopamine in the behavioral effects of caffeine in animals and humans. *Pharmacology, Biochemistry and Behavior, 57*(3), 533-541.

Gattaz, W. F., Abrahão, A. L., & Foccacia, R. (2004). Childhood meningitis, brain maturation and the risk of psychosis. *European Archives of Psychiatry and Clinical Neuroscience, 254*(1), 23-26.

Gesch, C. B., Hammond, S. M., Hampson, S. E., Eves, A., & Crowder, M. J. (2002). Influence of supplementary vitamins, minerals and essential fatty acids on the antisocial behaviour of young adult prisoners. Randomised, placebo-controlled trial. *The British Journal of Psychiatry, 181*, 22-28.

Giannini, A. J., Nakoneczie, A. M., Melemis, S. M., Ventresco, J., & Condon, M. (2000). Magnesium oxide augmentation of verapamil maintenance therapy in mania. *Psychiatry Research, 93*(1), 83-87.

Göder, R., Boigs, M., Braun, S., Friege, L., Fritzer, G., Aldenhoff, J. B., & Hinze-Selch, D. (2004). Impairment of visuospatial memory is associated with decreased slow wave sleep in schizophrenia. *Journal of Psychiatric Research, 38*(6), 591-599.

Göder, R., Fritzer, G., Gottwald, B., Lippmann, B., Seeck-Hirschner, M., Serafin, I., & Aldenhoff, J. B. (2008). Effects of olanzapine on slow wave sleep, sleep spindles and sleep-related memory consolidation in schizophrenia. *Pharmacopsychiatry, 41*(3), 92-99.

Godfrey, P. S., Toone, B. K., Carney, M. W., Flynn, T. G., Bottiglieri, T., Laundy, M., . . . Reynolds, E. H. (1990). Enhancement of recovery from psychiatric illness by methylfolate. *Lancet, 336*(8712), 392-395.

Goldman, M., Tandon, R., DeQuardo, J. R., Taylor, S. F., Goodson, J., & McGrath, M. (1996). Biological predictors of 1-year outcome in schizophrenia in males and females. *Schizophrenia Research, 21*(2), 65-73.

Gordon, C., & Galloway, T. (2008). *Review of Findings on Chronic Disease Self-Management Program (CDSMP) Outcomes: Physical, Emotional & Health-Related Quality of Life, Healthcare Utilization and Costs.* Centers for Disease Control and Prevention and National Council on Ageing.

Granon, S., Passetti, F., Thomas, K. L., Dalley, J. W., Everitt, B. J., & Robbins, T. W. (2000). Enhanced and impaired attentional performance after infusion of D1 dopaminergic receptor agents into rat prefrontal cortex. *The Journal of Neuroscience, 20*(3), 1208-1215.

Grimson, M. (2011, June 21). *High Caffeine Use Linked to Psychotic Symptoms.* Retrieved from ABC News: http://www.abc.net.au/news/2011-06-21/high-caffeine-use-linked-to-psychotic-symptoms/2766144

Groat, R. D., & Mackenzie, T. B. (1980). The appearance of mania following intravenous calcium replacement. *The Journal of Nervous and Mental Disease, 168*(9), 562-563.

Grossman, P., Jannsen, K. H., & Vaitl, D. (1986). *Cardiorespiratory and Cardiosomatic Psychophysiology.* New York: Plenum Press.

Gustafsson, P. A., Birberg-Thornberg, U., Duchén, K., Landgren, M., Malmberg, K., Pelling, H., . . . Karlsson, T. (2010). EPA supplementation improves teacher-rated behaviour and oppositional symptoms in children with ADHD. *Acta Paediatrica, 99*(10), 1540-1549.

Gutkowska, J., Jankowski, M., Mukaddam-Daher, S., & McCann, S. M. (2000). Oxytocin is a cardiovascular hormone. *Brazilian Journal of Medical and Biological Research, 33*(6), 625-633.

Haddad, P. M. (2004). Antipsychotics and diabetes: Review of non-prospective data. *The British Journal of Psychiatry. Supplement, 47*, S80-86.

Hansen, V., Jacobsen, B. K., & Arnesen, E. (2001). Cause-specific mortality in psychiatric patients after deinstitutionalisation. *The British Journal of Psychiatry, 179*, 438-443.

Hedges, D. W., Woon, F. L., & Hoopes, S. P. (2009). Caffeine-induced psychosis. *CNS Spectrums, 14*(3), 127-129.

Hibbard, J. H., & Collins, A. (2008). *Long Term Conditions Collaborative: Improving Self Management Support.* Retrieved from Scotland.gov.uk: http://www.scotland.gov.uk/Resource/Doc/274194/00 82012.pdf

Hibbard, J. H., Collins, A., & Baker, L. (2008). Clinician activation: Physician beliefs about patient self-management. *Background paper for the*

Commonwealth Fund and the Nuffield Trust - 9th International Meeting on Quality of Health Care.

Hibbeln, J. R., & Davis, J. M. (2009). Considerations regarding neuropsychiatric nutritional requirements for intakes of omega-3 highly unsaturated fatty acids. *Prostaglandins, Leukotrienes, and Essential Fatty Acids, 81*(2-3), 179-186.

Hirayama, S., Hamazaki, T., & Terasawa, K. (2004). Effect of docosahexaenoic acid-containing food administration on symptoms of attention-deficit/hyperactivity disorder - a placebo-controlled double-blind study. *European Journal of Clinical Nutrition, 58*(3), 467-473.

Hoffer, A. (1999). *Orthomolecular Treatment for Schizophrenia.* Lincolnwood: Keats.

Hofstetter, J. R., Lysaker, P. H., & Mayeda, A. R. (2005). Quality of sleep in patients with schizophrenia is associated with quality of life and coping. *BMC Psychiatry, 5*, 13.

Horne, J. A. (1993). Human sleep, sleep loss and behaviour. Implications for the prefontal cortex and psychiatric disorder. *The British Journal of Psychiatry, 162*, 413-419.

Houben, J. M., Mercken, E. M., Ketelslegers, H. B., Bast, A., Wouters, E. F., Hageman, G. J., & Schols, A. M. (2009). Telomere shortening in chronic obstructive pulmonary disease. *Respiratory Medicine, 103*(2), 230-236.

Howard, J. S. (1975). Folate deficiency in psychiatric practice. *Psychosomatics, 16*(3), 112-115.

Howe, L. (2012, December 13). *Press Release - More Choice in Mental Health.* Retrieved from GOV.UK: https://www.gov.uk/government/news/more-choice-in-mental-health

Huang, M. H., Friend, D. S., Sunday, M. E., Singh, K., Haley, K., Austen, K. F., . . . Smith, T. W. (1996). An intrinsic adrenergic system in mammalian heart. *The Journal of Clinical Investigation, 98*(6), 1298-1303.

Hunter, R., Jones, M., Jones, T. G., & Matthews, D. M. (1967). Serum B12 and folate concentrations in mental patients. *The British Journal of Psychiatry, 113*, 1291-1295.

Improving Chronic Illness Care. (2003). *The Chronic Care Model: Self-Management Support.* Retrieved from Improving Chronic Illness Care: http://www.improvingchroniccare.org/index.php?p=Self-Management_Support&s=22

Institute of HeartMath. (2001). *Science of the Heart: Exploring the Role of the Heart in Human Performance.* Boulder Creek: Institute of HeartMath. Retrieved from Beyond the Barriers.

Isen, A. M. (1998). On the relationship between affect and creative problem solving. In S. W. Russ, *Affect, Creative Experience, and Psychological Adjustment* (pp. 3-17). Philadelphia: Brunner/Mazel.

Isenring, E. (2008). Nutrition and mental health research: Where to from here? *Nutrition and Dietetics, 65*(1), 4-5.

Javitt, D. C., Silipo, G., Cienfuegos, A., Shelley, A. M., Bark, N., Park, M., . . . Zukin, S. R. (2001). Adjunctive high-dose glycine in the treatment of schizophrenia. *The International Journal of Neuropsychopharmacology, 4*(4), 385-391.

Javitt, D. C., Zylberman, I., Zukin, S. R., Heresco-Levy, U., & Lindenmayer, J. P. (1994). Amelioration of negative symptoms in schizophrenia by glycine. *The American Journal of Psychiatry, 151*(8), 1234-1236.

Källström, B., & Nylöf, R. (1969). Vitamin-B12 and folic acid in psychiatric disorders. *Acta Psychiatrica Scandinavica, 45*(2), 137-152.

Kantrowitz, J. T., Oakman, E., Bickel, S., Citrome, L., Spielman, A., Silipo, G., . . . Javitt, D. C. (2010). The importance of a good night's sleep; An open-label trial of the sodium salt of gamma-hydroxybutyric acid in insomnia associated with schizophrenia. *Schizophrenia Research, 120*(1-3), 225-226.

Kawasaki, H., & Iwamuro, S. (2008). Potential roles of histones in host defense as antimicrobial agents. *Infectious Disorders Drug Targets, 8*(3), 195-205.

Kentsch, M., Lawrenz, R., Ball, P., Gerzer, R., & Müller-Esch, G. (1992). Effects of atrial natriuretic factor on anterior pituitary hormone secretion in normal man. *The Clinical Investigator, 70*(7), 549-555.

Khan, Z. U., & Muly, E. C. (2011). Molecular mechanisms of working memory. *Behavioural Brain Research, 219*(2), 329-341.

Koch, T., Jenkin, P., & Kralik, D. (2004). Chronic illness self-management: Locating the 'self'. *Journal of Advanced Nursing, 48*(5), 484-492.

Koolhaas, J. M., Bartolomucci, A., Buwalda, B., de Boer, S. F., Flügge, G., Korte, S. M., . . . Fuchs, E. (2011). Stress revisited: A critical evaluation of the stress concept. *Neuroscience and Biobehavioral Reviews, 35*(5), 1291-1301.

Koponen, H., Rantakallio, P., Veijola, J., Jones, P., Jokelainen, J., & Isohanni, M. (2004). Childhood central nervous system infections and risk for schizophrenia. *European Archives of Psychiatry and Clinical Neuroscience, 254*(1), 9-13.

Kruger, A. (1996). Chronic psychiatric patients' use of caffeine: Pharmacological effects and mechanisms. *Psychological Reports, 78*(3 Pt 1), 915-923.

Kruger, A. (2000). Schizophrenia: Recovery and hope. *Psychiatric Rehabilitation Journal, 24*, 29-37.

Kyriacou, C. P., & Hastings, M. H. (2010). Circadian clocks: Genes, sleep, and cognition. *Trends in Cognitive Sciences, 14*(6), 259-267.

Lacey, B. C., & Lacey, J. I. (1978). Two-way communication between the heart and the brain. Significance of time within the cardiac cycle. *The American Psychologist, 33*(2), 99-113.

Lacey, J. I., & Lacey, B. C. (1970). Some autonomic-central nervous system interrelationships. In P. Black, *Physiological Correlates of Emotion* (pp. 205-227). New York: Academic Press.

Lafourcade, M., Larrieu, T., Mato, S., Duffaud, A., Sepers, M., matias, I., . . . Manzoni, O. J. (2011). Nutritional omega-3 deficiency abolishes endocannabinoid-mediated neural functions. *Nature Neuroscience, 14*(3), 345-350.

Lakhan, S. E., & Vieira, K. F. (2008). Nutritional therapies for mental disorders. *Nutrition Journal, 7*, 2.

Lamb, N. (2012, November 12). *NHS shakeup tackles disparity between mental and physical health services.* Retrieved from The Guardian: http://www.guardian.co.uk/society/2012/nov/12/nhs-shakeup-disparity-mental-health

Lamb, N. (2012, December 13). *Press Release - More Choice in Mental Health.* Retrieved from GOV.UK: https://www.gov.uk/government/news/more-choice-in-mental-health

Lambeth and Southwark Mind. (n.d.). *What Is Self-Management?* Retrieved June 2013, from Lambeth and Southwark Mind:

http://lambethandsouthwarkmind.org.uk/wp-content/uploads/2012/12/self-mang-participant-leaflet.pdf

Lara, D. R. (2010). Caffeine, mental health, and psychiatric disorders. *Journal of Alzheimer's Disease, 20 Suppl 1*, S239-248.

Lasevoli, F., Latte, G., Avvisati, L., Sarappa, C., Aloj, L., & de Bartolomeis, A. (2012). The expression of genes involved in glucose metabolism is affected by N-methyl-D-aspartate receptor antagonism: A putative link between metabolism and an animal model of psychosis. *Journal of Neuroscience Research, 90*(9), 1756-1767.

Laughlin, S. B. (2004). The implications of metabolic energy requirements for the representation of information in neurons. In M. S. Gazzaniga, *The Cognitive Neurosciences* (pp. 187-196). Cambridge: MIT Press.

Lawn, S., & Battersby, M. (2009). Skills for person-centred care: Health professionals supporting chronic condition prevention and self-management. In H. M. D'Cruz, S. W. Jacobs, & A. Schoo, *Knowledge-in-Practice in the Caring Professions: Multi-Disciplinary Perspectives* (pp. 161-192). Farnham: Ashgate Publishing.

Lawn, S., Battersby, M. W., Pols, R. G., Lawrence, J., Parry, T., & Urukalo, M. (2007). The mental health expert patient: Findings from a pilot study of a generic chronic condition self-management programme for people with mental illness. *The International Journal of Social Psychiatry, 53*(1), 63-74.

Lawrence, D. M., Holman, C. D., Jablensky, A. V., & Hobbs, M. S. (2003). Death rate from ischaemic heart disease in Western Australian psychiatric patients 1980-1998. *The British Journal of Psychiatry, 182*, 31-36.

Leiderman, E., Zylberman, I., Zukin, S. R., Cooper, T. B., & Javitt, D. C. (1996). Preliminary investigation of high-dose oral glycine on serum levels and negative symptoms in schizophrenia: An open-label trial. *Biological Psychiatry, 39*(3), 213-215.

Leitner, Z. A., & Church, I. C. (1956). Nutritional studies in a mental hospital. *Lancet, 270*(6922), 565-567.

Lichtermann, D., Ekelund, J., Pukkala, E., Tanskanen, A., & Lönngvist, J. (2001). Incidence of cancer among persons with schizophrenia and their relatives. *Archives of General Psychiatry, 58*(6), 573-578.

Lipton, K., Mailman, R., & Numeroff, C. (1979). Vitamins, megavitamin therapy and the nervous system. In R. Wurtman, & W. Wurtman, *Nutrition and the Brain* (pp. 183-264). New York: Raven Press.

Lloyd, J., & Wait, S. (2006). *Integrated Care: A Guide for Policymakers.* London: Alliance for Health & the Future.

Lorig, K. R., Sobel, D. S., Stewart, A. L., Brown, B. W., Bandura, A., Ritter, P., . . . Holman, H. R. (1999).

Evidence suggesting that a chronic disease self-management program can improve health status while reducing hospitalization: A randomized trial. *Medical Care, 37*(1), 5-14.

Lucas, P. B., Pickar, D., Kelsoe, J., Rapaport, M., Pato, C., & Hommer, D. (1990). Effects of the acute administration of caffeine in patients with schizophrenia. *Biological Psychiatry, 28*(1), 35-40.

Maas, J. W., Gleser, G. C., & Gottschalk, L. A. (1961). Schizophrenia, anxiety, and biochemical factors. The rate of oxidation of N, N-dimethyl-p-phenylenediamine by plasma and levels of serum copper and plasma ascorbic acid. *Archives of General Psychiatry, 4*, 109-118.

MacKarness, R. (1976). *Eating Dangerously*. New York: Harcourt Brace Jovanovich.

Mahadik, S. P., Pillai, A., Joshi, S., & Foster, A. (2006). Prevention of oxidative stress-mediated neuropathology and improved clinical outcome by adjunctive use of a combination of antioxidants and omega-3 fatty acids in schizophrenia. *International Review of Psychiatry, 18*(2), 199-131.

Manoach, D. S., & Stickgold, R. (2009). Does abnormal sleep impair memory consolidation in schizophrenia. *Frontiers in Human Neuroscience, 3*, 21.

Manoach, D. S., Cain, M. S., Vangel, M. G., Khurana, A., Goff, D. C., & Stickgold, R. (2004). A failure of sleep-dependent procedural learning in chronic, medicated schizophrenia. *Biological Psychiatry, 56*(12), 951-956.

Manoach, D. S., Thakkar, K. N., Stroynowski, E., Ely, A., McKinley, S. K., Wamsley, E., . . . Stickgold, R. (2010). Reduced overnight consolidation of procedural learning in chronic medicated schizophrenia is related to specific sleep stages. *Journal of Psychiatric Research, 44*(2), 112-120.

Martin, J. L., Jeste, D. V., & Ancoli-Israel, S. (2005). Older schizophrenia patients have more disrupted sleep an circadian rhythms than age-matched comparison subjects. *Journal of Psychiatric Research, 39*(3), 251-259.

Martin, J., Jeste, D. V., Caliguiri, M. P., Patterson, T., Heaton, R., & Ancoli-Israel, S. (2001). Actigraphic estimates of circadian rhythms and sleep/wake in older schizophrenia patients. *Schizophrenia Research, 47*(1), 77-86.

Mathieu, G., Denis, S., Lavialle, M., & Vancassel, S. (2008). Synergistic effects of stress and omega-3 fatty acid deprivation on emotional response and brain lipd composition in adult rats. *Prostaglandins, Leukotrienes, and Essential Fatty Acids, 78*(6), 391-401.

McCraty, R. (2000). Psychophysiological coherence: A link between positive emotions, stress reduction, performance and health. *Eleventh International Congress on Stress.* Mauna Lani Bay.

McCraty, R. (2003). *The Energetic Heart: Bioelectromagnetic Interactions Within and Between People.* Boulder Creek: Institute of HeartMath.

McCraty, R. (2003b). *Heart-Brain Neurodynamics: The Making of Emotions.* Boulder Creek: Institute of HeartMath.

McCraty, R., & Tamasino, D. (2006). Emotional stress, positive emotions, and psychophysiological coherence. In B. B. Arnetz, & R. Ekman, *Stress in Health and Disease* (pp. 342-365). Weinheim: Wiley-VCH.

McCraty, R., Atkinson, M., Tiller, W. A., Rein, G., & Wakins, A. D. (1995). The effects of emotions on short-term power spectrum analysis of heart rate variability. *The American Journal of Cardiology, 76*(14), 1089-1093.

McCraty, R., Atkinson, M., Tomasino, D., & Bradley, R. T. (2006). *The Coherent Heart.* Boulder Creek: Institute of HeartMath.

McCraty, R., Bradley, R. T., & Tomasino, D. (2004-2005, December-February). The Resonant Heart. *Shift: At the Frontiers of Consciousness.*

McEvoy, M. (2013, February 6). *Bacteria & the Brain: The Powerful Behavior-Modifying Effects of the Gut.* Retrieved from Metabolic Healing: http://metabolichealing.com/key-integrated-functions-of-your-body/gut/bacteria-and-the-brain-the-powerful-behavior-modifying-effects-of-the-gut/

McManamy, M. C., & Schube, P. G. (1936). Caffeine intoxication: Report of a case the symptoms of which amounted to a psychosis. *New England Journal of Medicine, 215*, 616-620.

McNay, E. C., McCarty, R. C., & Gold, P. E. (2001). Fluctuations in brain glucose concentration during behavioral testing: Dissocations between brain areas and between brain and blood. *Neurobiology of Learning and Memory, 75*, 325-327.

Mental Health Foundation. (2012, August 16). *New Self-Management Guidance Launched to Help People with Long Term Mental Health Problems.* Retrieved from Mental Health Foundation: http://www.mentalhealth.org.uk/our-news/news-archive/2012/184202/

Mental Health Foundation. (n.d.). *Self-Management.* Retrieved from Mental Health Foundation: http://mentalhealth.org.uk/help-information/mental-health-a-z/S/self-management/

Mental Health Wiki. (2010). *Circadian Rhythms.* Retrieved from Mental Health Wiki: http://www.mentalhealthwiki.org/Circadian_rhythms

Mikkelsen, E. J. (1978). Caffeine and schizophrenia. *The Journal of Clinical Psychiatry, 39*(9), 732-736.

Miller, J. G. (1978). *Living Systems.* New York: McGraw-Hill.

Moyer, K. E. (1975). Allergy & aggression: The physiology of violence. *Psychology Today*, 77-79.

Müller, N., & Schwarz, M. J. (2007). The immunological basis of glutamatergic disturbance in schizophrenia: Towards an integrated view. *Journal of Neural Transmission. Supplementum*(72), 269-280.

Müller, N., & Schwarz, M. J. (2007b). The immune-mediated alteration of serotonin and glutamate: Towards an integrated view of depression. *Molecular Psychiatry, 12*(11), 988-1000.

Murphy, D. A., Thompson, G. W., Ardell, J. L., McCraty, R., Stevenson, R. S., Sangalang, V. E., . . . Armour, J. A. (2000). The heart reinnervates after transplantation. *The Annals of Thoracic Surgery, 69*(6), 1769-1781.

Murphy, D. L., Baker, M., Goodwin, F. K., Miller, H., Kotin, J., & Bunney, W. E. (1974). L-tryptophan in affective disorders: Indoleamine changes and differential clinical effects. *Psychopharmacologia, 34*(1), 11-20.

Murray, G., & Harvey, A. (2010). Circadian rhythms and sleep in bipolar disorder. *Bipolar Disorders, 12*(5), 459-472.

Murray, R. (2012, November). *The Abandoned Illness.* Retrieved from Rethink: http://www.rethink.org/media/514088/TSC_executive _summary_14_nov.pdf

Myers, E., Startup, H., & Freeman, D. (2011). Cognitive behavioural treatment of insomnia in individuals with persistent persecutory delusions: A pilot trial. *Journal of Behavior Therapy and Experimental Psychiatry, 42*(3), 330-336.

National Institute of General Medical Sciences. (2012, November). *Circadian Rhythms Fact Sheet.* Retrieved from National Institute of General Medical Sciences: http://www.nigms.nih.gov/Education/Factsheet_Circ adianRhythms.htm

Nawrot, P., Jordan, S., Eastwood, J., Rotstein, J., Hugenholtz, A., & Feeley, M. (2003). Effects of caffeine on human health. *Food Additives and Contaminants, 20*(1), 1-30.

Naylor, C., Parsonage, M., McDaid, D., Knapp, M., Fossey, M., & Galea, A. (2012). *Long-Term Conditions and Mental Health: The Cost of Co-morbidities.* London: The King's Fund.

Naylor, G. J., & Smith, A. H. (1981). Vanadium: A possible aetiological factor in manic depressive illness. *Psychological Medicine, 11*(2), 249-256.

Nehlig, A., Daval, J. L., & Debry, G. (1992). Caffeine and the central nervous system: Mechanisms of action, biochemical, metabolic and psychostimulant effects. *Brain Research. Brain Research Reviews, 17*(2), 139-170.

Nemets, H., Nemets, B., Apter, A., Bracha, Z., & Belmaker, R. H. (2006). Omega-3 treatment of childhood depression: A controlled, double-blind pilot study. *The American Journal of Psychiatry, 163*(6), 1098-1100.

O'Brien, S. M., Scully, P., Scott, L. V., & Dinan, T. G. (2006). Cytokine profiles in bipolar affective disorder: Focus on acutely ill patients. *Journal of Affective Disorders, 90*(2-3), 263-167.

Opstad, K. (1994). Circadian rhythm of hormones is extinguished during prolonged physical stress, sleep and energy deficiency in young men. *European Journal of Endocrinology, 131*(1), 56-66.

Packer, L. (1999). *The Antioxidant Miracle: Put Lipoic Acid, Pycnogenol, and Vitamins E and C to Work for You.* Canada: John Wiley & Sons.

Paluska, S. A. (2003). Caffeine and exercise. *Current Sports Medicine Reports, 2*(4), 213-219.

Pappas, S. (2012, December 18). *Suicide Attempts Linked to Inflammatory Chemical.* Retrieved from Live Science: http://www.livescience.com/25637-suicide-attempts-linked-inflammation.html

Pataracchia, R. J. (2002). *Nutritional Management of Schizophrenia.* Retrieved from International Guide to the World of Alternative Mental Health: http://www.alternativementalhealth.com/articles/nutritionschizophrenia.htm

Peedicayil, J. (2007). The role of epigenetics in mental disorders. *The Indian Journal of Medical Research, 126,* 105-111.

Peet, M. (2003). Eicosapentaenoic acid in the treatment of schizophrenia and depression: Rationale and preliminary double-blind clinical trial results. *Prostaglandins, Leukotrienes and Essential Fatty Acids, 69*(6), 477-485.

Peet, M. (2004). Nutrition and schizophrenia: Beyond omega-3 fatty acids. *Prostaglandins, Leukotrienes and Essential Fatty Acids, 70*(4), 417-422.

Peet, M. (2004b). International variations in the outcome of schizophrenia and the prevalence of depression in relation to national dietary practices: An ecological analysis. *The British Journal of Psychiatry, 184*, 404-408.

Perkins, R. (2013). *Can mental health services as we know them really support recovery?* Retrieved from Scottish Recovery: https://www.google.co.uk/url?sa=t&rct=j&q=&esrc=s&source=web&cd=2&cad=rja&ved=0CEkQFjAB&url=http%3A%2F%2Fwww.scottishrecovery.net%2FDownload-document%2F365-National-Gathering-2013-Dr-Rachel-Perkins-OBE-Presentation.html&ei=Bsy1UfS5JdCz0QWHr4HoCw&usg=AFQjC

Peters, Z. (2012, December 13). *Turning Point responds to the government's proposals for greater patient involvement.* Retrieved from Turning Point: http://www.turning-point.co.uk/news-and-events/news/turning-point-

responds-to-the-government%E2%80%99s-proposals-
for-greater-patient-involvement.aspx

Pfeiffer, C. C., & Braverman, E. R. (1979). Folic acid and
vitamin b12 therapy for the low-histamine, high
copper biotype of schizophrenia. In M. I. Botez, & E.
N. Reynolds, *Folic Acid in Neurology, Psychiatry and
Internal Medicine*. New York: Raven Press.

Phelan, M., Stradins, L., & Morrison, S. (2001). Physical health
of people with severe mental illness. *BMJ (Clinical
Research Ed.), 322*(7284), 443-444.

Poulos, J., Stoddard, D., & Carron, K. (1976). *Alcoholism, Stress
and Hypoglycemia*. Santa Cruz: Davis Publishing.

Prange, A. J., Wilson, I. C., Lynn, C. W., Alltop, L. b., &
Stikeleather, R. A. (1974). L-tryptophan in mania.
Contribution to a permissive hypothesis of affective
disorders. *Archives of General Psychiatry, 30*(1), 56-62.

Ptak, C., & Petronis, A. (2010). Epigenetic approaches to
psychiatric disorders. *Dialogues in Clinical
Neuroscience, 12*(1), 25-35.

Purcell, S. M., Consortium, I. S., Wray, N. R., Stone, J. L.,
Visscher, P. M., O'Donovan, M. C., . . . Sklar, P. (2009).
Common polygenic variation contributes to risk of
schizophrenia and bipolar disorder. *Nature, 460*(7256),
748-752.

Puri, B. K., Richardson, A. J., Horrobin, D. F., Easton, T.,
Saeed, N., Oatridge, A., . . . Bydder, G. M. (2000).

Eicosapentaenoic acid treatment in schizophrenia associated with symptom remission, normalisation of blood fatty acids, reduced neuronal membrane phospholipid turnover and structural brain changes. *International Journal of Clinical Practice, 54*(1), 57-63.

Quinn, C. (2009). Supplements for mental health. *Mental Health Practice, 12*(9), 26-27.

Randich, A., & Gebhart, G. F. (1992). Vagal afferent modulation of nociception. *Brain Research. Brain Research Reviews, 17*(2), 77-99.

Rein, G., Atkinson, M., & McCraty, R. (1995). The psysiological and psychological effects of compassion and anger. *Journal of Advancement in Medicine, 8*(2), 87-105.

Reivich, M., & Alavi, A. (1983). Positron emission tomographic studies of local cerebral glucose metabolism in humans in physiological and pathological conditions. *Advances in Metabolic Disorders, 10*, 135-176.

Repper, J., & Perkins, R. (2003). *Social Inclusion and Recovery*. London: Balliere Tindall.

Rethink Mental Illness. (2012). *Schizophrenia Commission Report.*

Rethink Mental Illness. (n.d.). *What Is Recovery? - Treatment & Support*. Retrieved June 2013, from Rethink Mental Illness: http://www.rethink.org/living-with-mental-illness/recovery/what-is-recovery/treatment-support

Reynolds, E. H. (1975). Letter: Folate-responsive
    schizophrenia. *Lancet, 2*(7926), 189-190.

Richardson, A. J. (2003). The role of omega-3 fatty acids in
    behaviour, cognition and mood. *Scandinavian Journal
    of Nutrition, 47*(2), 92-98.

Richardson, A. J., & Montgomery, P. (2005). The Oxford-
    Durham study: A randomized, controlled trial of
    dietary supplementation with fatty acids in children
    with developmental coordination disorder. *Pediatrics,
    115*(5), 1360-1366.

Richardson, A. J., & Puri, B. K. (2002). A randomized double-
    blind, placebo-controlled study of the effects of
    supplementation with highly unsaturated fatty acids
    on ADHD-related symptoms in children with specific
    learning difficulties. *Progress in
    Neuropsychopharmacology & Biological Psychiatry,
    26*(2), 233-239.

Richardson, A. J., Easton, T., & Puri, B. K. (2000). Red cell and
    plasma fatty acid changes accompanying symptom
    remission in a patient with schizophrenia treated
    with eicosapentaenoic acid. *European
    Neuropsychopharmacology, 10*(3), 189-193.

Richardson, A. J., Easton, T., Gruzelier, J. H., & Puri, B. K.
    (1999). Laterality changes accompanying symptom
    remission in schizophrenia following treatment with
    eicosapentaenoic acid. *International Journal of
    Psychophysiology, 34*(3), 333-339.

Rix, K. J., Ditchfield, J., Freed, D. L., Goldberg, D. P., & Hillier, V. F. (1985). Food antibodies in acute psychoses. *Psychological Medicine, 15*(2), 347-354.

Robbins, T. W. (2002). The 5-choice serial reaction time task: Behavioural pharmacology and functional neurochemistry. *Psychopharmacology, 163*(3-4), 362-380.

Roffman, J. L., Lamberti, J. S., Achtyes, E., Macklin, E. A., Galendez, G. C., Raeke, L. H., . . . Goff, D. C. (2013). Randomized multicenter investigation of folate plus vitamin B12 supplementation in schizophrenia. *JAMA Psychiatry, 70*(5), 481-489.

Rogers, P. J., Appleton, K. M., Kessler, D., Peters, T. J., Gunnell, D., Hayward, R. C., . . . Ness, A. R. (2008). No effect of n-3 long-chain polyunsaturated fatty acid (EPA and DHA) supplementation on depressed mood and cognitive function: A randomised controlled trial. *The British Journal of Nutrition, 99*(2), 421-431.

Rudin, D. O. (1981). The major psychoses and neuroses as omega-3 essential fatty acid deficiency syndrome: Substrate pellagra. *Biological Psychiatry, 16*(9), 837-850.

Ruxton, C. H., & Derbyshire, E. (2009). Latest evidence on omega-3 fatty acids and health. *Nutrition & Food Science, 39*(4), 423-438.

Sacks, W., Esser, A. H., Feitel, B., & Abbott, K. (1989). Acetazolamide and thiamine: An ancillary therapy for chronic mental illness. *Psychiatry Research, 28*(3), 279-288.

Sandman, C. A., Walker, B. B., & Berka, C. (1982). Influence of afferent cardiovascular feedback on behavior and the cortical evoked potential. In J. T. Cacioppo, & R. E. Petty, *Perpectives in Cardiovascular Psychophysiology* (pp. 189-222). New York: The Guildford Press.

Schauss, A. G. (1984). Nutrition and antisocial behaviour. *International Clinical Nutrition Review, 4*(4), 172-177.

Schauss, A. G., & Simonsen, C. E. (1979). Critical analysis of the diets of chronic juvenile offenders: Part I. *Journal of Orthomolecular Psychiatry, 8*(3), 149-157.

Schorah, C. J., Morgan, D. B., & Hullin, R. P. (1983). Plasma vitamin C concentrations in patients in a psychiatric hospital. *Human Nutrition. Clinical Nutrition, 37*(6), 447-452.

Schweizer, U., Bräuer, A. U., Köhrle, J., Nitsch, R., & Savaskan, N. E. (2004). Selenium and brain function: A poorly recognised liaison. *Brain Research. Brain Research Reviews, 45*(3), 164-178.

Scott, W. H., Coyne, K. M., Johnson, M. M., Lausted, C. G., Sahota, M., & Johnson, A. T. (2002). Effects of caffeine on performance of low intensity tasks. *Perceptual and Motor Skills, 94*(2), 521-532.

Seamans, J. K., & Yang, C. R. (2004). The principal features and mechanisms of dopamine modulation in the prefrontal cortex. *Progress in Neurobiology, 74*(1), 1-58.

Seisjo, B. K. (1978). *Brain Energy Metabolism.* Chichester: John Wiley & Sons.

Selvadurai, E. (2012, August 1). *Mild mental illness 'raises risk of premature death'.* Retrieved from BBC News Health: http://www.bbc.co.uk/news/health-19061271

Shaul, P. W., Farrell, M. K., & Maloney, M. J. (1984). Caffeine toxicity as a cause of acute psychosis in anorexia nervosa. *The Journal of Pediatrics, 105*(3), 493-495.

Shen, W. W., & D'Souza, T. C. (1979). Cola-induced psychotic organic brain syndrome. A case report. *Rocky Mountain Medical Journal, 76*(6), 312-313.

Shepherd, G., Boardman, J., & Slade, M. (2008, March). *Making Recovery A Reality.* Retrieved from Sainsbury Centre for Mental Health: http://www.centreformentalhealth.org.uk/pdfs/Making_recovery_a_reality_policy_paper.pdf

Shi, J., Levinson, D. F., Duan, J., Sanders, A. R., Zheng, Y., Pe'er, I., . . . Gejman, P. V. (2009). Common variants on chromosome 6p22.1 are associated with schizophrenia. *Nature, 460*(7256), 753-757.

Sinn, N., & Bryan, J. (2007). Effect of supplementation with polyunsaturated fatty acids and micronutrients on

learning and behavior problems associated with child
ADHD. *Journal of Developmental and Behavioral
Pediatrics, 28*(2), 82-91.

Slade, M. (2009). *100 Ways to Support Recovery: A Guide for
Mental Health Professionals. Rethink Recovery Series:
Volume 1.* Retrieved from Mental Health Recovery:
http://www.mentalhealthrecovery.com/recovery-
resources/documents/100_ways_to_support_recovery
1.pdf

Slade, M. (2009). *Personal Recovery and Mental Illness: A Guide
for Mental Health Professionals.* New York: Cambridge
University Press.

Spangler, R., Wittkowski, K. M., Goddard, N. L., Avena, N. M.,
Hoebel, B. G., & Leibowitz, S. F. (2004). Opiate-like
effects of sugar on gene expression in reward areas of
the rat brain. *Brain Research Molecular Brain
Research, 124*(2), 134-142.

Stefansson, H., Ophoff, R. A., Steinberg, S., Andreassen, O. A.,
Cichon, S., Rujescu, D., . . . Collier, D. A. (2009).
Common variants conferring risk of schizophrenia.
Nature, 460(7256), 744-747.

Stevens, L., Zhang, W., Peck, L., Kuczek, T., Grevstad, N.,
Mahon, A., . . . Burgess, J. R. (2003). EFA
supplementation in children with inattention,
hyperactivity, and other disruptive behaviors. *Lipids,
38*(10), 1007-1021.

Stickgold, R. (2005). Sleep-dependent memory consolidation. *Nature, 437*(7063), 1272-1278.

Ströhle, A., Kellner, M., Holsboer, F., & Wiedemann, K. (1998). Atrial natriuretic hormone decreases endocrine response to a combined dexamethasone-corticotropin-releasing hormone test. *Biological Psychiatry, 43*(5), 371-375.

Suboticanec, K. (1986). Vitamin C status in schizophrenia. *Bibliotheca Nutritio Dieta*(38), 173-181.

Sullivan, E. L., Grayson, B., Takahashi, D., Robertson, N., Maier, A., Bethea, C. L., . . . Grove, K. L. (2010). Chronic consumption of a high fat diet during pregnancy causes perturbations in the serotonergic system and increased anxiety-like behaviour in non-human primate offspring. *The Journal of Neuroscience, 30*(10), 3826-30.

Sullivan, R. M. (2004). Hemispheric asymmetry in stress processing in rat prefrontal cortex and the role of mesocortical dopamine. *Stress, 7*(2), 131-143.

Svensson, T. H., & Thorén, P. (1979). Brain noradrenergic neurons in the locus coeruleus: Inhibition by blood volume load through vagal afferents. *Brain Research, 172*(1), 174-178.

Swain, A., Soutter, V., Loblay, R., & Truswell, A. S. (1985). Salicylates, oligoantigenic diets, and behaviour. *Lancet, 2*(8445), 41-42.

Swerdlow, N. R., van Bergeijk, D. P., Bergsma, F., Weber, E., & Talledo, J. (2009). The effects of memantine of prepulse inhibition. *Neuropsychopharmacology, 34*(7), 1854-1864.

Tchirkov, A., & Lansdorp, P. M. (2003). Role of oxidative stress in telomere shortening in cultured fibroblasts from normal individuals and patients with ataxia-telangiectasia. *Human Molecular Genetics, 12*(3), 227-232.

Telegdy, G. (1994). The action of ANP, BNP and related peptides on motivated behavior in rats. *Reviews in the Neurosciences, 5*(4), 309-315.

The Franklin Institute. (2004). *Nourish - Micronutrients - Maintaining the Oxygen Balance in Your Brain.* Retrieved from The Franklin Institute: http://www.fi.edu/learn/brain/micro.html

The Healing Partnership. (n.d.). *Dr. Bonnet Discusses Pyroluria.* Retrieved from The Healing Partnership: http://www.thehealingpartnership.org/pdf/pyroluria_handout.pdf

The Mental Health Foundation. (2006, June). *Feeding Minds: The impact of food on mental health.* Retrieved from Mental Health: http://www.mentalhealth.org.uk/content/assets/PDF/publications/Feeding-Minds.pdf

The Schizophrenia Comission. (2012, November). *The Abandoned Illness.* Retrieved from Rethink:

http://www.rethink.org/media/514088/TSC_executive
_summary_14_nov.pdf

The Wellesley Institute. (2009, January). *Mental Health "Recovery": Users and Refusers*. Retrieved from Wellesley Institute: http://wellesleyinstitute.com/files/Mental_Health%20_Recovery.pdf

Thompson, K. M., Wonderlich, S. A., Crosby, R. D., & Mitchell, J. E. (1999). The neglected link between eating disturbances and aggressive behavior in girls. *Journal of the American Academy of Child and Adolescent Psychiatry, 38*(10), 1277-1284.

Tiller, W. A., McCraty, R., & Atkinson, M. (1996). Cardiac coherence: A new, noninvasive measure of autonomic nervous system order. *Alternative Therapies in Health and Medicine, 2*(1), 52-65.

Trevizol, F., Benvegnú, D. M., Barcelos, R. C., Boufleur, N., Dolci, G. S., Müller, L. G., . . . Bürger, M. E. (2011). Comparative study between n-6, trans and n-3 fatty acids on repeated amphetamine exposure: A possible factor for the development of mania. *Pharmacology, Biochemistry, and Behavior, 97*(3), 560-565.

Tripuraneni, B. R. (1990). Treatment of lithium-induced polyuria with potassium: A political study. *American Psychiatric Association*, (p. 84). New York.

Vaddadi, K. S., Courtney, P., Gilleard, C. J., Manku, M. S., & Horrobin, D. F. (1989). A double-blind trial of essential fatty acid supplementation in patients with tardive dyskinesia. *Psychiatry Research, 27*(3), 313-323.

Vaisman, N., Kaysar, N., Zaruk-Adasha, Y., Pelled, D., Brichon, G., Zwingelstein, G., & Bodennec, J. (2008). Correlation between changes in blood fatty acid composition and visual sustained attendtion performance in children with inattention: Effect of dietary n-3 fatty acids containing phospholipids. *The American Journal of Clinical Nutrition, 87*(5), 1170-1180.

van der Heijden, F. M., Fekkes, D., Tuinier, S., Sijben, A. E., Kahn, R. S., & Verhoeven, W. M. (2005). Amino acids in schizophrenia: Evidence for lower tryptophan availability during treatment with atypical antipsychotics? *Journal of Neural Transmission, 112*(4), 577-585.

Van Dongen, H. P., Maislin, G., Mullington, J. M., & Dinges, D. F. (2003). The cumulative cost of additional wakefulness: Dose-response effects on neurobehavioral functions and sleep physiology from chronic sleep restriction and total sleep deprivation. *Sleep, 26*(2), 117-126.

van Kammen, D. P., Yao, J. K., & Goetz, K. (1989). Polyunsaturated fatty acids, prostaglandins, and schizophrenia. *Annals of the New York Academy of Sciences, 559*, 411-423.

Velázquez, A., & Bourges, H. (1984). Genetic factors in nutrition. Orlando: Academic Press.

Virkkunen, M. (1983). Insulin secretion during the glucose tolerance test in antisocial personality. *The British Journal of Psychiatry, 142*, 598-604.

Voigt, R. G., Llorente, A. M., Jensen, C. L., Fraley, J. K., Berretta, M. C., & Heird, W. C. (2001). A randomized, double-blind, placebo-controlled trial of docosahexaenoic acid supplementation in children with attention-deficit/hyperactivity disorder. *The Journal of Pediatrics, 139*(2), 189-196.

Vollmar, A. M., Lang, R. E., Hänze, J., & Schulz, R. (1990). A possible linkage of atrial natriuretic peptide to the immune system. *American Journal of Hypertension, 3*(5 Pt 1), 408-411.

Warner, R. (2010). *Editorial: Does the scientific evidence support the recovery model?* Retrieved from The Psychiatrist: pb.rcpsych.org/content/34/1/3.full.pdf

Watfa, G., Dragonas, C., Brosche, T., Dittrich, R., Sieber, C. C., Alecu, C., . . . Nzietchueng, R. (2011). Study of telomere length and different markers of oxidative stress in patients with Parkinson's disease. *The Journal of Nutrition, Health & Ageing, 15*(4), 277-281.

Watson, G. (1979). *Personality, Strength and Psyco-Chemical Energy.* New York: Harper & Row.

Weiss, V. (1978). From memory span to the quantum mechanics of intelligence. *Personality and Individual Differences, 7*, 737-749.

Wesensten, N. J., Belenky, G., Kautz, M. A., Thorne, D. R., Reichardt, R. M., & Balkin, T. J. (2002). Maintaining alertness and performance during sleep deprivation: modafinil versus caffeine. *Psychopharmacology, 159*(3), 238-247.

Wichers, M. C., Myin-Germeys, I., Jacobs, N., Peeters, F., Kenis, G., Derom, C., . . . van Os, J. (2007). Evidence that moment-to-moment variation in positive emotions buffer genetic risk for depression: A momentary assessment twin study. *Acta Psychiatrica Scandinavica, 115*(6), 451-457.

Wikgren, M., Maripuu, M., Karlsson, T., Nordfjäll, K., Bergdahl, J., Hultdin, J., . . . Norrback, K. F. (2012). Short telomeres in depression and the general population are associated with a hypocortisolemic state. *Biological Psychiatry, 71*(4), 294-300.

Wirleitner, B., Neurauter, G., Schröcksnadel, K., Frick, B., & Fuchs, D. (2003). Interferon-gamma-induced conversion of tryptophan: Immunologic and neuropsychiatric aspects. *Current Medicinal Chemistry, 10*(16), 1581-1591.

Wittchen, H. U., Jacobi, F., Rehm, J., Gustavsson, A., Svensson, M., Jönsson, B., . . . Steinhausen, H. C. (2011). The size and burden of mental disorders and other disorders of the brain in Europe 2010. *European Neuropsychopharmacology, 21*(9), 655-679.

Wolpert, S. (2008, July 9). *Scientists learn how what you eat affects your brain - and those of your kids.* Retrieved

from UCLA Newsroom:
http://newsroom.ucla.edu/portal/ucla/scientists-learn-how-food-affects-52668.aspx

Woodward, D. J., Moises, H. C., Waterhouse, B. D., Yeh, H. H., & Cheun, J. E. (1991). Modulatory actions of norepinephrine on neural circuits. *Advances in Experimental Medicine and Biology, 287*, 193-208.

World Federation for Mental Health. (n.d.). *Can Anxiety Increase My Risk for Heart Disease?* Retrieved June 2013, from Sharecare: http://www.sharecare.com/question/can-anxiety-risk-heart-disease

Wulff, K., & Joyce, E. (2011). Circadian rhythms and cognition in schizophrenia. *The British Journal of Psychiatry, 198*(4), 250-252.

Wulff, K., Joyce, E., Middleton, B., Dijk, D. J., & Foster, R. G. (2006). The suitability of actigraphy, diary data, and urinary melatonin profiles for quantitative assessment of sleep disturbances in schizophrenia: A case report. *Chronobiology International, 23*(1-2), 485-495.

Wulff, K., Porcheret, K., Cussans, E., & Foster, R. G. (2009). Sleep and circadian rhythm disturbances: Multiple genes and multiple phenotypes. *Current Opinion in Genetics & Development, 19*(3), 237-246.

Yamashita, H., Mori, K., Okamoto, Y., Morinobu, S., & Yamawaki, S. (2004). Effects of changing from typical to atypical antipsychotic drugs on subjective sleep quality in patients with schizophrenia in a Japanese population. *The Journal of Clinical Psychiatry, 65*(11), 1525-1530.

Yang, C., & Winkelman, J. W. (2006). Clinical significance of sleep EEG abnormalities in chronic schizophrenia. *Schizophrenia Research, 82*(2-3), 251-260.

Yao, J. K., Magan, S., Sonel, A. F., Gurklis, J. A., Sanders, R., & Reddy, R. D. (2004). Effects of omega-3 fatty acid on platelet serotonin responsivity in patients with schizophrenia. *Prostaglandins, Leukotrienes and Essential Fatty Acids, 71*(3), 171-176.

Yudofsky, S. C., Silver, J. M., & Hales, R. E. (1990). Pharmacologic management of aggression in the elderly. *The Journal of Clinical Psychiatry, 51 Suppl,* 22-28.

Zhang, M., Zhao, Z., He, L., & Wan, C. (2010). A meta-analysis of oxidative stress markers in schizophrenia. *Science China. Life Sciences, 53*(1), 112-124.

Zubin, J., & Spring, B. (1977). Vulnerability - A new view of schizophrenia. *Journal of Abnormal Psychology, 86*(2), 103-126.

Zuckerman, L., & Weiner, I. (2005). Maternal immune activation leads to behavioral and pharmacological changes in the adult offspring. *Journal of Psychiatric Research, 39*(3), 311-323.

GLOSSARY

DISORDERS

Alzheimer's Disease: A progressive disorder that gradually destroys a person's memory and ability to learn, reason, make judgments, communicate and carry out daily activities. Individuals with more advanced stages of Alzheimer's disease may also experience changes in personality and behaviour such as anxiety, suspiciousness or agitation, as well as delusions or hallucinations. The disease usually starts in middle or old age, beginning with memory loss concerning recent events and spreading to memory loss concerning events that are more distant.

Anxiety Disorders: Chronic feelings of overwhelming anxiety and fear, unattached to any obvious source, that can grow progressively worse if not treated. The anxiety is often accompanied by physical symptoms such as sweating, cardiac disturbances, diarrhoea or dizziness. Generalised anxiety disorder, panic disorder, agoraphobia, obsessive-compulsive disorder and posttraumatic stress disorder are considered anxiety disorders.

Bipolar Disorder: Also known as manic-depressive illness. A serious illness that causes shifts in a person's mood, energy and ability to function. Dramatic mood swings can move from "high" feelings of extreme euphoria or irritability to depression, sometimes with periods of normal moods in between. Manic episodes may include such behaviours as prolonged periods without sleep or uncontrolled shopping. Each episode of mania or depression can last for hours, weeks or several months.

Dementia: A group of diseases that cause a permanent decline of a person's ability to think, reason and manage his/her own life. Dementia is caused by biological processes within the brain that damage brain cells.

Depression: In psychiatry, a disorder marked especially by sadness, inactivity, difficulty with thinking and concentration, a significant increase or decrease in appetite and time spent sleeping, feelings of dejection and hopelessness and sometimes suicidal thoughts or attempts to commit suicide. While standing alone as a mental illness, depression also can be experienced in other disorders such as bipolar disorder. Depression can range from mild to severe.

Generalised Anxiety Disorder (GAD): Characterised by excessive uncontrollable worry about everyday things. The chronic worrying can affect daily functioning and cause physical symptoms, filling an individual's days with tension even though there is little or nothing to provoke it. Unlike a phobia, Generalised Anxiety Disorder is not triggered by a specific object or situation. Individuals with this disorder are always anticipating disaster, often worrying excessively about health, money, family or work. In addition to chronic worry, symptoms may include trembling, muscular aches, insomnia, abdominal upsets, dizziness and irritability.

Obsessive-Compulsive Disorder: A disorder in which individuals are plagued by persistent, recurring thoughts or obsessions that reflect exaggerated anxiety or fears. Typical obsessions include worry about being contaminated or fears of behaving improperly or acting violently. The obsessions may lead to the performance of ritual or routine compulsions such as washing hands, repeating phrases or hoarding.

Panic Disorder: An anxiety disorder in which individuals have feelings of terror that strike suddenly and repeatedly with no warning. Individuals cannot predict when an attack will occur and may develop intense anxiety between episodes, worrying when the next one will strike. Symptoms can include heart palpitations, chest pain or discomfort, sweating, trembling, tingling sensations, a feeling of choking, fear of dying, fear of losing control and feelings of unreality.

Parkinson's Disease: A progressive, neurodegenerative disease that occurs when the neurons within the brain responsible for producing the chemical dopamine becomes impaired or dies.

Schizophrenia: A psychotic disorder characterised by loss of contact with the environment, noticeable deterioration in the level of functioning in everyday life and disintegration of feeling, thought and conduct. Individuals with schizophrenia often hear internal voices not heard by others (hallucinations) or believe things that other people find absurd (delusions). The symptoms also may include disorganised speech and grossly disorganised or catatonic behaviour. Individuals with schizophrenia have marked impairment in social or occupational functioning.

Seasonal Affective Disorder (SAD): A form of depression occurring at certain seasons of the year, especially when the individual has less exposure to sunlight.

Social Anxiety Disorder: Also called social phobia. An anxiety disorder in which a person has an excessive and unreasonable fear of social situations. Anxiety (intense nervousness) and self-consciousness arise from a fear of being closely watched, judged, and criticised by others. The fear may be made worse by a lack of social skills or experience in social situations, and can build into a panic attack. People with anxiety disorder suffer from distorted thinking, including false beliefs about social situations and the negative opinions of others. As a result of the fear, the person endures certain social situations in extreme distress or may avoid them altogether.

A

Acetylcholine: A compound that occurs throughout the nervous system, in which it functions as a neurotransmitter.

Adenosine Triphosphate (ATP): A substance present in all living cells that provides energy for many metabolic processes and is involved in making RNA. It's the only usable form of energy in the body.

Adrenaline: See *Epinephrine.*

Agonist: A substance that initiates a physiological response when combined with a receptor.

Amino Acid: One of the 20 building blocks from which proteins are assembled. Isoleucine, leucine, lysine, phenylalanine, threonine, tryptophan, and valine are deemed 'essential' amino acids because the human body cannot make them and they must be obtained in the diet. Amino acids are sometimes taken orally in supplement form.

Amygdala: Located in the middle of the brain, this almond shaped complex of related nuclei is a critical processor area for the senses. Connected to the hippocampus, it plays a role in emotionally laden memories. It contains a huge number of opiate receptor sites implicated in rage, fear and sexual feelings.

Anabolic: Means 'building-up'. The phrase of metabolism in which simple substances are synthesised into the complex materials of living tissue.

Antagonist: Actively oppose; a substance that interferes with or inhibits the physiological action of another.

Antioxidant: A chemical compound or substance that inhibits oxidation or a substance, such as vitamin E, vitamin C, or beta carotene, thought to protect body cells from the damaging effects of oxidation.

Autonomic Nervous System (ANS): A part of the nervous system that regulates key involuntary functions of the body, including the activity of the heart muscle; the smooth muscles, including the muscles of the intestinal tract; and the glands.

Axon: The long portion of a neuron that conducts impulses away from the body of the cell. Also called nerve fibre.

B

Biochemical Individuality: The concept that the nutritional and chemical make-up of each person is unique and that dietary needs therefore vary from person to person.

Biochemical Pathway: The long chains of chemical reactions, catalysed by enzymes, that occur in all living cells, and take place in the normal operation of living systems.

C

Catabolic: The metabolic breakdown of complex molecules into simpler ones, often resulting in a release of energy.

Central Nervous System (CNS): Is comprised of the brain and spinal cord. The CNS receives sensory information from the peripheral nervous system (PNS) and controls the body's responses.

Circadian Rhythms: Physical, mental and behavioural changes that follow a roughly 24-hour cycle, responding primarily to light and darkness in an organism's environment. They are found in most living things, including animals, plants and many tiny microbes. The study of circadian rhythms is called chronobiology.

Co-morbidity: In general, the existence of two or more illnesses – whether physical or mental – at the same time in a single individual. The term can also refer to the coexistence of mental illness and substance abuse.

Collaboration: Is both a process and an outcome in which shared interest or conflict that cannot be addressed by any single individual is addressed by key stakeholders. A key stakeholder is any party directly influenced by the actions others take to solve a complex problem. The collaborative process involves a synthesis of different perspectives to better understand complex problems. A collaborative outcome is the development of integrative solutions that go beyond an individual vision to a productive resolution that could not be accomplished by any single person or organization.

D

Delusion: A belief that is false, fanciful or derived from deception. In psychiatry, a false belief strongly held in spite of evidence that it is not true, especially as a symptom of a mental illness.

Dendrites: The branch-like structures of neurons that extend from the cell body (soma). The dendrites receive neural impulses (electrical and chemical signals) from the axons of other neurons. The signal always travels in the same direction – the signal comes into the neuron through the dendrites, through the soma, to the axon, and then out the terminal buttons to the dendrites of the next neuron. In this way information travels all around your body going from neuron to neuron.

Detoxification: The metabolic process by which toxins are changed into less toxic or more readily excretable substances.

Diabetes Mellitus: Or simply diabetes, is a condition in which a person has high blood sugar, either because the pancreas no longer produces enough insulin (type 1 diabetes), or because the cells stop responding to the insulin that is produced (type 2 diabetes).

DNA Methylation: The modification of a strand of DNA after it is replicated, in which a methyl (CH3) group is added to any cytosine molecule that stands directly before a guanine molecule in the same chain. Since methylation of cytosines in particular regions of a gene can cause that gene's suppression, DNA methylation is one of the methods used to regulate the expression of genes.

Dopamine: Is both a neurotransmitter and a neurohormone produced in multiple areas of the brain. As a hormone it is often associated with pleasant experiences. As a neurotransmitter it transmits signals associated with concentration and motor skills. Conditions such as Parkinson's disease and schizophrenia are associated with an interruption in the brain's production of dopamine.

Dopaminergic: Pertaining to the action of dopamine or to neural or metabolic pathways in which it functions as a transmitter.

E

Endogenous: Growing or originating from within an organism.

Enzyme: A protein formed by the body that acts as a catalyst to cause a certain desired reaction. Enzymes are very specific; each enzyme is designed to initiate a specific response with a specific result.

Epigenetics: The study of the chemical modification of specific genes or gene-associated proteins of an organism. Epigenetic modifications can define how the information in genes is expressed and used by cells.

Epinephrine: (Also adrenaline) is a hormone and a neurotransmitter having many functions in the body – regulateing heart rate, blood vessel and air passage diameters, and metabolic shifts. It is a crucial component of the fight-or-flight response of the sympathetic nervous system (SNS).

Essential Fatty Acids (EFAs): Fatty acids that humans and other animals must ingest because the body requires them for good health but cannot synthesize them. The term "essential fatty acid" refers to fatty acids required for biological processes but does not include the fats that only act as fuel.

Essential Nutrient: A nutrient required for normal body functioning that either cannot be synthesized by the body at all, or cannot be synthesized in amounts adequate for good health (e.g. niacin, choline), and thus must be obtained from a dietary source.

Exogenous: Originating from outside an organism

F

Free Radical: An atom or group of atoms that has at least one unpaired electron and is therefore unstable and highly reactive. In animal tissues, free radicals can damage cells and are believed to accelerate the progression of cancer, cardiovascular disease, and age-related diseases.

G

Gene Expression: The process by which a gene's coded information is translated into the structures present and operating in the cell (either proteins or RNAs).

Glial Cell: A supportive cell in the CNS. Unlike neurons, glial cells do not conduct electrical impulses. The glial cells surround neurons and provide support for and insulation between them. Glial cells are the most abundant cell types in the CNS.

Glucagon: A hormone produced by the pancreas that stimulates an increase in blood sugar levels, thus opposing the action of insulin.

Glycaemic Foods: "Causing glucose (sugar) in the blood". High glycaemic foods have a Glycaemic Index (GI) of 60 or above, and are applied only to carbohydrates. Foods that fall into this category are usually processed foods that contain high amounts of sugar, white flour products and artificial sweeteners.

Glycation: A reaction that takes place when simple sugar molecules, such as fructose or glucose, become attached to proteins or lipid fats without the moderation of any enzyme. This results in the formation of rogue molecules known as Advanced Glycation Endproducts (AGEs).

Glycolysis: The process in cell metabolism by which carbohydrates and sugars, especially glucose, are broken down, producing ATP and pyruvic acid.

H

Homeostasis: The ability to maintain a constant internal environment in response to environmental changes. It is a unifying principle of biology. The nervous and endocrine systems control homeostasis in the body through feedback mechanisms involving various organs and organ systems. Examples of homeostatic processes in the body include temperature control, pH balance, water and electrolyte balance, blood pressure, and respiration.

Homocysteine: An amino acid found in blood. There is now considerable evidence that homocysteine may prove to be a useful marker for risk of heart attacks, since elevated levels have been detected in people with coronary artery disease.

Hypoglycaemia: Occurs when the level of glucose in the blood is lower than it should be.

Hypothalamic-Pituitary-Adrenal (HPA) Axis: A complex set of interactions between the hypothalamus, the pituitary gland and the adrenal or suprarenal glands (at the top of each kidney). The HPA Axis helps regulate things such as temperature, digestion, immune system, mood, sexuality and energy usage. It's also a major part of the system that controls your reaction to stress, trauma and injury.

Hypothalamus: A region of the forebrain below the thalamus that coordinates both the autonomic nervous system and the activity of the pituitary.

I

Insulin: Is a hormone produced by the pancreas that helps the body use glucose for energy.

Insulin Resistance: Occurs when the body doesn't respond as well to the insulin that the pancreas is making and glucose is less able to enter the cells. People with insulin resistance may or may not go on to develop type 2 diabetes.

Immune System: The body system, made up of many organs and cells, that defends the body against infection, disease and foreign substances. The immune system is often stimulated in specific ways to fight cancer cells. A system (including the thymus, bone marrow and lymphoid tissues) that protects the body from foreign substances and pathogenic organisms by producing the immune response. A system that provides a defence mechanism to organism, providing defensive measures against antigens which would prove harmful to the organism.

Inflammation: One of the most common ways the immune system reacts to any type of bodily injury. Inflammation can occur in joints, on the skin, within organs, and so forth. It is characterized by redness, warmth, swelling and pain.

M

Macronutrients: Nutrients that the body uses in relatively large amounts, such as proteins, carbohydrates and fats.

Mania: Excitement manifested by mental and physical hyperactivity, disorganisation of behaviour, and elevation of mood.

Metabolism: The chemical processes occurring within a living cell or organism that are necessary for the maintenance of life. In metabolism some substances are broken down to yield energy for vital processes while other substances, necessary for life, are synthesised.

Metabolic Syndrome: A combination of medical disorders that, when occurring together, increase the risk of developing cardiovascular disease and diabetes.

Micronutrients: These are in our diets, but in very small amounts. These can be found in vitamins, minerals and trace elements. Micronutrients, like water, do not provide energy, however they are still needed in adequate amounts to ensure that our bodily cells function properly.

Myelin: A fatty substance that covers neurons. Around your neurons is a myelin sheath (a layer of myelin) that helps increase the speed at which information can travel on the neurons.

N

Negative Feedback: A feedback that tends to stabilise a process by reducing its rate or output when its effects are too great.

Neuroendocrine: Relating to, or involving, the interation between the nervous system and the hormones of the endocrine glands.

Neuropeptide Y (NPY): A 36-amino acid peptide that acts as a neurotransmitter in the brain and in the ANS.

Noradrenaline: See *Norepinephrine.*

Norepinephrine: (Also noradrenaline) is a catecholamine with multiple roles including as a hormone and a neurotransmitter. As a neurotransmitter, norepinephrine is released from the sympathetic neurons affecting the heart, increasing the rate of contractions. As a stress hormone, it affects parts of the brain – such as the amygdala – where attention and responses are controlled. Along with epinephrine, norepinephrine underlies the fight-or-flight response.

Neuron: A specialised cell transmitting nerve impulses; a nerve cell.

Neurotransmitter: A chemical that is released from a nerve cell which thereby transmits an impulse from a nerve cell to another nerve, muscle, organ, or other tissue. A neurotransmitter is a messenger of neurologic information from one cell to another.

Nutrient: A source of nourishment, especially an ingredient in a food.

Nutritional Therapy: Combines science (biochemistry and nutrition) with naturopathy (natural, drug-free medicine) in order to return the patient to a state of good health. Nutritional therapy is holistic because it is designed to treat the body as a whole – curing the causes of problems, not just the symptoms, as is too often the case in conventional medicine.

O

Obesity: A medical condition in which excess body fat has accumulated to the extent that it may have an adverse effect on health.

Olanzapine: A atypical antipsychotic drug used to treat schizophrenia; to control manic episodes of bipolar disorder (manic-depressive disorder); or to treat dementia related to Alzheimer's disease.

Omega-3: Refers to a group of three fats called A-Linolenic Acid (ALA), found in plant oils; Eicosapentaenoic Acid (EPA), and Docosahexaenoic Acid (DHA), both commonly found in marine oils. These are essential polyunsaturated fats; they are not made by the human body and must be obtained from food.

Omega-6: Refers to a family of unsaturated fatty acids found in nuts, poultry, cereals and most vegetable oils. A high proportion of omega-6 to omega-3 fat in the diet shifts the physiological state in the tissues toward the pathogenesis of many diseases: prothrombotic, proinflammatory and proconstrictive. A diet with a ratio of 4 to 1 or lower omega-6 to omega-3 is thought to be optimal.

Opioid: Possessing some properties characteristic of opiate narcotics but not derived from opium – such as a synthetic nartoic that resembles the naturally occurring opiates, or any substance that binds to or otherwise affects the opiate receptors on the surface of the cell. For example, medications that relieve pain.

Orthomolecular: Relating to or aimed at restoring the optimal concentrations and functions at the molecular level of the substances (e.g., vitamins) normally present in the body.

Oxidation: The interaction between oxygen molecules and all the different substances they may contact – from metal to living tissue. Technically, however, with the discovery of electrons, oxidation came to be more precisely defined as the loss of at least one electron when two or more substances interact.

Oxidative Stress: An imbalance between the production of reactive oxygen and a biological system's ability to readily detoxify the reactive intermediates or easily repair the resulting damage.

P

Paranoia: Unfounded or exaggerated distrust of others, sometimes reaching delusional proportions. Paranoid individuals constantly suspect the motives of those around them, and believe that certain individuals, or people are "out to get them."

Parasympathetic Nervous System (PSNS): A part of the ANS. Its main function is to conserve/restore the body's energy. For example, sending signals to slow the heart rate and breathing, or speed up the digestive tract in order to process calories and save energy.

Peripheral Nervous System (PNS): That portion of the nervous system that is outside the brain and spinal cord.

Peripheral Neuropathy: A problem with the functioning of the nerves outside the spinal cord. Symptoms of peripheral neuropathy may include numbness, weakness, burning pain (especially at night), and loss of reflexes.

Positive Feedback: A feedback that tends to magnify a process or increase its output.

Psychoactive: Affecting mind or behaviour.

Psychosis: A serious mental disorder characterised by defective or lost contact with reality, often with hallucinations or delusions, causing deterioration of normal social functioning.

R

Recovery: A process by which people who have a mental illness are able to work, learn and participate fully in their communities. For some individuals, recovery is the ability to live a fulfilling and productive life despite a disability. For others, recovery implies the reduction or complete remission of symptoms.

S

Selective Serotonin Reuptake Inhibitors (SSRI): A class of antidepressants that act within the brain to increase the amount of serotonin, a chemical nerves use to send messages to one another (neurotransmitter). Neurotransmitters are released by one nerve and taken up by other nerves. Those that are not taken up by other nerves are taken up by the same nerve that released them, a process called reuptake. By inhibiting reuptake, SSRIs allow more serotonin to be taken up by other nerves.

Self-Management: Transferring the focus from treating a condition or illness to enabling people to live with it in the long term. Within the context of mental ill health, the focus does not have to be on a diagnosis or a particular illness; rather it can be on how to respond to the obstacles faced by the individual, whether these are viewed through a neurological, biochemical, psychological, social or spiritual lens.

Sensorimotor: Of, relating to, or combining the functions of the sensory and motor activities.

Serious Mental Illness (SMI): A diagnosable mental disorder found in individuals aged 18 years and older. The disorder is so severe and long lasting it seriously interferes with a person's ability to take part in major life activities.

Serotonin: A naturally occurring chemical in the brain (a neurotransmitter) that is responsible, in part, for regulating brain functions such as mood, appetite, sleep, and memory.

Sympathetic Nervous System (SNS): A part of the ANS which is responsible for mobilising the body's fight-or-flight response. It is, however, constantly active at a basic level to maintain homeostasis.

Synapse: A junction between two nerve cells, consisting of a minute gap across which impulses pass by diffusion of a neurotransmitter.

T

Telomere: The end of a chromosome. The ends of chromosomes are specialized structures that are involved in the replication and stability of DNA molecules. A telomere is a length of DNA that is made up of a repeating sequence of six nucleotide bases (TTAGGG).

Tryptophan: A type of amino acid that is essential (not naturally produced by the body and must be provided by the diet). Like all amino acids, tryptophan acts as a building block in protein biosynthesis. In addition it acts as a biochemical precursor for serotonin, niacin and auxin (a phytohormone).

W

Withdrawal Symptoms: Feelings of discomfort, distress and intense craving for a substance that occur when use of the substance is stopped. These symptoms occur because the body had become metabolically adapted to the substance. The withdrawal symptoms can range from mild discomfort to actual life threatening.

INDEX